ADULT CONSEQUENCES OF PEDIATRIC ORTHOPAEDIC CONDITIONS

EDITED BY

PETER D. PIZZUTILLO, MD
PROFESSOR OF ORTHOPAEDIC SURGERY AND PEDIATRICS
DREXEL UNIVERSITY COLLEGE OF MEDICINE
DIRECTOR OF ORTHOPAEDIC SURGERY
ST. CHRISTOPHER'S HOSPITAL FOR CHILDREN
PHILADELPHIA, PENNSYLVANIA

MARTIN J. HERMAN, MD
ASSOCIATE PROFESSOR OF ORTHOPEDIC SURGERY AND PEDIATRICS
DREXEL UNIVERSITY COLLEGE OF MEDICINE
ST. CHRISTOPHER'S HOSPITAL FOR CHILDREN
PHILADELPHIA, PENNSYLVANIA

SERIES EDITOR

HENRY D. CLARKE, MD
CONSULTANT, DEPARTMENT OF ORTHOPEDIC SURGERY
ASSOCIATE PROFESSOR OF ORTHOPEDIC SURGERY, COLLEGE OF MEDICINE
MAYO CLINIC
PHOENIX, ARIZONA

LIBRARY

College of Physicians and Surgeons
of British Columbia

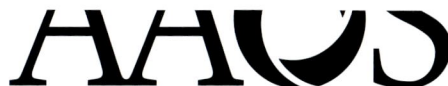

AAOS
AMERICAN ACADEMY OF ORTHOPAEDIC SURGEONS

AAOS

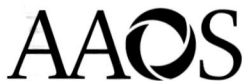

AMERICAN ACADEMY OF ORTHOPAEDIC SURGEONS

**Adult Consequences of Orthopaedic
Pediatric Conditions**

Published 2013 by the
American Academy of Orthopaedic Surgeons
6300 North River Road
Rosemont, IL 60018

ISSN 2328-272X
ISBN
978-0-89203-954-8
Printed in the USA

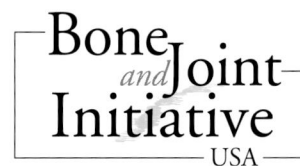

Bone *and* Joint Initiative
USA

CONTRIBUTORS

Joshua M. Abzug, MD
Fellow, Pediatric Upper Extremity
Department of Orthopaedics
Shriners Hospitals for Children—
  Philadelphia
St. Christopher's Hospital for Children
Philadelphia, Pennsylvania

Todd J. Albert, MD
Professor and Chair
Department of Orthopaedics
Thomas Jefferson University
Philadelphia, Pennsylvania

Wen Chao, MD
Orthopaedic Attending
Department of Orthopaedic Surgery
University of Pennsylvania Health System
Philadelphia, Pennsylvania

Mark L. Dumonski, MD
Spine Fellow
Department of Orthopaedics
Thomas Jefferson University
Philadelphia, Pennsylvania

Jeremy S. Frank, MD
Fellow, Pediatric Sports Medicine
Division of Sports Medicine
Boston Children's Hospital
Boston, Massachusetts

Martin J. Herman, MD
Associate Professor of Orthopedic
  Surgery and Pediatrics
Drexel University College of Medicine
St. Christopher's Hospital for Children
Philadelphia, Pennsylvania

Norman A. Johanson, MD
Chairman, Department of Orthopaedic
  Surgery
Drexel University College of Medicine
Philadelphia, Pennsylvania

Mininder S. Kocher, MD, MPH
Associate Director, Division of Sports
  Medicine
Associate Professor of Orthopedic Surgery
Department of Orthopedic Surgery
Boston Children's Hospital
Boston, Massachusetts

Scott H. Kozin, MD
Orthopaedic Surgeon
Hand/Upper Extremity
Department of Orthopaedics
Shriners Hospitals for Children—
  Philadelphia
Philadelphia, Pennsylvania

James J. McCarthy, MD
Division Director
Department of Orthopedic Surgery
Cincinnati Children's Hospital
Cincinnati, Ohio

Lyle J. Micheli, MD
Director, Division of Sports Medicine
O'Donnell Family Professor of Orthopedic
  Sports Medicine
Department of Orthopedic Surgery
Boston Children's Hospital
Boston, Massachusetts

CONTRIBUTORS (CONT.)

Michael B. Millis, MD
Director, Adolescent and Young Adult
  Hip Unit
Department of Orthopedic Surgery
Boston Children's Hospital
Boston, Massachusetts

Martin J. Morrison III, MD
Fellow, Department of Orthopedic Surgery
The Children's Hospital of Philadelphia
Philadelphia, Pennsylvania

Eduardo N. Novais, MD
Fellow, Adolescent and Young Adult
  Hip Unit
Department of Orthopedic Surgery
Boston Children's Hospital
Boston, Massachusetts

Peter D. Pizzutillo, MD
Professor of Orthopaedic Surgery and
  Pediatrics
Drexel University College of Medicine
Director of Orthopaedic Surgery
St. Christopher's Hospital for Children
Philadelphia, Pennsylvania

Satheesh Kumar Ramineni, MD
Staff Orthopaedic Surgeon
Surgery Service
Oklahoma City VA Medical Center
Oklahoma City, Oklahoma

Matthew W. Squire, MD, MS
Department of Orthopedics and
  Rehabilitation
University of Wisconsin
Madison, Wisconsin

CONTENTS

PREFACE

Recent advances in medical care have resulted in improved quality of life, prolonged years of activity, and increased longevity for patients with orthopaedic conditions. These changes apply not only to able-bodied individuals but also to those with physical challenges. As a result, the numbers of adults who present to general orthopaedic surgeons with complaints stemming from childhood conditions and injuries are increasing.

Children and adolescents with musculoskeletal problems have long been diligently treated and followed to skeletal maturity by pediatric orthopaedic surgeons. The adult sequelae of these orthopaedic problems have not been well described and the transition to care under general orthopaedic surgeons has been difficult.

The objective of this monograph, *Adult Consequences of Pediatric Orthopaedic Conditions*, is to provide the orthopaedic surgeon caring for the adult patient with authoritative, current recommendations from the literature that are based on the experience of leading clinicians in both pediatric and adult orthopaedic subspecialties. This monograph is unique because its population-based focus differs from that of condition-based publications.

This monograph was inspired by the care, research, and dedication of G. Dean MacEwen, MD, who provided comprehensive, lifelong care for children with orthopaedic conditions. Dr. MacEwen has been the model and inspiration for several generations of pediatric orthopaedic surgeons throughout the world. His progressive thinking and broad-based approach to clinical care are well known and have been emulated by many clinicians.

We would like to thank our contributing authors for their thoughtful contributions to this monograph. We also thank the members of the AAOS publications department, specifically Hans Koelsch, PhD, director; Lisa Claxton Moore, managing editor; Steven Kellert, senior editor; and Rachel Winokur, publications assistant, for their guidance and efforts in producing a monograph that provides unique, need-to-know information to orthopaedic surgeons who continually strive to improve patient care.

Peter D. Pizzutillo, MD
Martin J. Herman, MD
Editors

CHAPTER 1

ISTHMIC SPONDYLOLISTHESIS AND SCOLIOSIS

MARK L. DUMONSKI, MD

TODD J. ALBERT, MD

INTRODUCTION

Spondylolisthesis is the condition in which a vertebral body is translated forward relative to the vertebral body below it. The etiologies associated with this pathologic process were originally outlined in the Wiltse-Newman five-part classification published in 1976.[1] Of the five types, isthmic spondylolisthesis is by far the most common in the pediatric population. Spondylolysis is a defect in the pars interarticularis and is often the cause of isthmic spondylolisthesis in children. Spondylolysis without associated spondylolisthesis may be a cause of back pain in the pediatric population.

Many patients with spondylolisthesis and spondylolysis are asymptomatic, and thus the true incidence of these conditions is unknown. Fredrickson et al[2] published an informative natural history study in 1984. The authors prospectively followed 500 first-grade children and noted a 4.4% incidence of spondylolysis at age 6 years, which increased to 6% in adulthood. Spondylolysis has an increased incidence in the Eskimo population (54% in adults),[3] in males (about twice that of females),[4] and in first-degree relatives of identified patients.[5] Spondylolysis has a significantly higher incidence in athletes[6,7] and it has not been reported in nonambulatory patients,[8] which suggests that upright posture and the stress imparted to the posterior elements of the vertebrae by the lumbar musculature may play a significant role in the development of a spondylolytic defect.

Scoliosis is generally defined as a coronal curvature of the spine greater than 10°. In 1955, Shands and Eisberg[9] reported on 50,000 minifilm radiographs of patients screened for tuberculosis and determined a prevalence of scoliosis of 1.9%. In 1982, a study by Lonstein et al[10] was the largest study conducted defining the prevalence of scoliosis in the pediatric population. Over a 7-year period, 1,473,697 students were screened; the overall reported prevalence of scoliosis was 1.1%. Although numerous theories regarding the etiology of scoliosis have been described, the underlying pathogenesis of adolescent idiopathic scoliosis (AIS) remains unclear, as

Dr. Albert or an immediate family member serves as a board member, owner, officer, or committee member of the American Academy of Orthopaedic Surgeons, the American Orthopaedic Association, the Cervical Spine Research Society, the Council for Value in Spine Care, and the Scoliosis Research Society; has received royalties from DePuy, a Johnson & Johnson company; serves as a paid consultant to or is an employee of DePuy, a Johnson & Johnson company; has stock or stock options held in Bioassets, Biomerix, Breakaway Imaging, Crosstree, Gentis, International Orthopaedic Alliance, Invuity, Paradigm Spine, PIONEER, Reville Consortium, and Vertech; and has received nonincome support (such as equipment or services), commercially derived honoraria, or other non–research-related funding (such as paid travel) from United Healthcare. Neither Dr. Dumonski nor any immediate family member has received anything of value from or has stock or stock options held in a commercial company or institution related directly or indirectly to the subject of this chapter.

the term implies. Genetics, however, does appear to play a role. Supporting evidence includes very high concordance rates of scoliosis among monozygotic twins,[11] a significantly increased incidence of scoliosis in daughters born to mothers with scoliosis,[12] and chromosomal links to genes that may be responsible for its pathogenesis.[13-15]

Commonly Used Childhood Interventions

Most cases of spondylolysis and spondylolisthesis are asymptomatic; therefore, other etiologies of pain (for example, diskitis, abdominal or pelvic conditions) should be investigated before instituting a treatment plan. The initial treatment of spondylolysis and spondylolisthesis is generally nonsurgical; the exceptions are for a progressive slip greater than 50% or the presence of objective neurologic impairment. Treatment goals include the elimination of pain, an increase in spinal mobility, treatment of hamstring contractures, and return to sports and routine daily activities. These goals are accomplished with activity modification and physical therapy. Contraction of the posterior paraspinal musculature is theorized to be a contributing factor; therefore, excessive lordotic posturing (spinal extension) should be avoided. Physical therapy should focus on flexion-based core muscle strengthening and treatment of associated hamstring contracture.

Bracing may be instituted if symptoms persist or the degree of slip increases despite activity modification and physical therapy. When the spondylolytic defect is due to an acute injury, bracing is a component of the initial treatment plan. In these situations, an antilordotic lumbosacral orthosis is worn full time for 3 to 6 months in conjunction with the aforementioned nonsurgical measures. With an acute injury, maximum immobilization is obtained by adding a leg extension to the lumbosacral orthosis. As symptoms lessen, use of the brace may be reduced to part-time wear, and ultimately discontinued. With the resolution of symptoms and restoration of strength and flexibility, the patient may gradually return to all prior activities without restriction.

Surgical treatment is recommended if at least 6 months of nonsurgical treatment has failed to resolve symptoms, if the slip is greater than 50% at presentation, if the slip has progressed since initial presentation, or if a neurologic deficit develops at any point. A detailed discussion outlining the various surgical treatment strategies is outside the scope of this chapter; however, options include posterior spinal fusion, direct repair of the spondylolytic defect, and rarely, anterior interbody fusion. Other surgical considerations include foraminal decompression using instrumentation or autograft bone, surgical reduction of the slip, and determining which vertebral levels should be included in the fusion construct.

Treatment options for AIS include observation, bracing, and surgical intervention. Skeletally immature patients with curves greater than 20° and less than 50° and those who have documented curve progression greater than 5° in a given year are candidates for bracing. The brace used is usually a thoracolumbosacral orthosis. The brace is worn full time, but it may be removed for showering, sports, and social activities. Weaning from brace wear is initiated once longitudinal spinal growth has ceased and the patient is at Risser grade 4 maturity. Weinstein et al[16] conducted a natural history study of skeletally mature patients with a mean follow-up of 40 years. Based on this study of mature patients, those curves exceeding 50° may still progress, and such patients may be candidates for surgical intervention.

Outcomes
Natural History

In 2003, Beutler et al[17] reported 45-year follow-up data for 30 children, age 6 years, with spondylolysis and spondylolisthesis in the only prospective long-term study of its kind. The results suggest a benign course. In no patient with a unilateral defect was spondylolisthesis diagnosed later. In patients with bilateral spondylolytic defects without a slip, 77% progressed to spondylolisthesis and none of the pars defects healed. Despite this, patients with bilateral L5 pars defects followed a clinical course similar to that of the general population. Patients who initially presented with spondylolisthesis and a mean slip of 11% progressed to a mean slip of 18% at final follow-up. No correlation was noted between slip progression and pain or function scores using a back pain questionnaire and the 36-Item Short Form Health Survey. In a similar 20-year follow-up study, Saraste[18] identified risk factors associated with long-term development of back pain that included a slip greater than 25%, a low lumbar index (in L5 spondylolysis), spondylolysis at the L4 level, and early disk degeneration.

As documented by Lonstein and Carlson[19] in 1984, approximately 23% of AIS curves that initially measured between 5° and 29° continued to progress. Factors that positively correlated with curve progression included presence of a double curve, greater curve magnitude, a lower Risser stage, and lack of menses. Once a patient reaches skeletal maturity, natural history studies indicate that a thoracic curve greater than 50° may progress throughout adulthood at a rate of 0.75° to 1.0° per year,[20] and a lumbar curve greater than 30° may progress at a rate of 0.4° per year. Other factors that correlated with a higher likelihood of lumbar curve progression included rotation and right-side curves. At long-term follow-up, patients with advanced scoliosis tended to have more back pain, and pulmonary function tended to be affected once the thoracic curve progressed beyond 100°.[21] For these reasons, surgical intervention is generally recommended in a patient with AIS and a thoracic curve exceeding 50°.

Results

Patients with spondylolysis and grade 1 or 2 spondylolisthesis do well with nonsurgical treatment.[22,23] A meta-analysis by Klein et al[23] identified a total of 665 patients who were treated nonsurgically, with an overall clinical success rate of 83.9%. Patients treated with a brace did not have better results than patients treated without a brace. Radiographic outcomes also were evaluated for a total of 847 defects, 28% of which healed. Substantially higher rates of healing were noted in unilateral versus bilateral defects and in defects that were acute versus chronic. Fujii et al[24] reported higher healing rates in patients with low-grade slips (<5%) versus higher-grade slips (≥5%). Children with symptomatic high-grade slips have significantly poorer results than children with spondylolysis or low-grade slips,[22] and symptom relief can be expected in only 10% of these patients. Surgical intervention is recommended in this patient population.

Lamberg et al[25] evaluated radiographic and clinical outcomes in 107 patients with spondylolysis and low-grade spondylolisthesis (<50%) who were surgically treated via posterior spondylodesis (29 patients) or posterolateral spondylodesis (78 patients). At a mean follow-up of 21 years, the mean Oswestry Disability Index score was 7.6 (minimal disability). At final follow-up, 14% of patients reported back pain either often or very often. Pseudarthrosis developed in 19% of patients, one half of whom were symptomatic and required additional surgery. Slip progression greater than 10° was noted in 10% of patients (mean preoperative slip, 34%). Oswestry Disability Index scores did not correlate with radiographic union, preoperative slip percentage, or postoperative slip percentage.

Molinari et al[26] reported on 32 consecutive patients with high-grade slips at a mean follow-up of 3 years. The patients had undergone posterior L4-S1 in situ fusion (group 1), posterior instrumented L4-S1 reduction and fusion (group 2), or posterior instrumented reduction followed by circumferential fusion (group 3). Despite the fact that slip angles were highest in group 3 and lowest in group 1, pseudarthrosis rates were highest in group 1 and lowest in group 3. Five of the six patients with symptomatic pseudarthrosis were subsequently treated with circumferential fusion (one refused treatment). All five had a solid fusion at final follow-up. The patient who refused surgery was being treated for chronic pain at final follow-up. Four patients (15%) had neurologic impairment following surgical reduction of spondylolisthesis. One patient's impairment resolved spontaneously; in one patient, foot drop spontaneously resolved, but unilateral extensor hallucis longus weakness was present at follow-up; in one patient, the neurologic deficit resolved after return to surgery and partial release of the surgical reduction; and one patient improved following intraoperative reversal of reduction and removal of instrumentation. Instrumentation failure occurred in 29% of patients in group 2 and in 16% of patients in group 3. Function, pain, and satisfaction scores were significantly increased in all groups at final follow-up.

Lehman et al[27] reported intermediate-term results of surgical treatment of 114 patients with AIS who were followed for at least 3 years. The main thoracic curve decreased from a mean of 59.2° preoperatively to 16.8° at final follow-up. The mean thoracolumbar/lumbar curve decreased from 44° preoperatively to 15° at final follow-up. No short-term or long-term neurologic complications were observed. A deep infection requiring additional surgeries developed in four (3.5%) patients, and two patients required an extension of their fusions from T12 to L4. Pulmonary function tests revealed significant improvements in forced vital capacity, forced expiratory volume in 1 second, and percentage of forced expiratory volume at final follow-up. The mean Scoliosis Research Society score was also significantly higher at final follow-up (76.5% preoperatively versus 83.0% postoperatively).

ADULT SEQUELAE
Presenting Symptoms
Most adult patients with spondylolysis and isthmic spondylolisthesis are asymptomatic. Even when the patient has a history of either spondylolysis or spondylolisthesis as a child, the patient's clinical course is likely to follow that of the general population.[17] Back pain is the most common symptom. Children with spondylolysis and isthmic spondylolisthesis exhibited earlier radiographic evidence of disk degeneration than children in the control group.[18] Therefore, whether the patient's back pain is related to a lytic defect or is a consequence of disk degeneration is unclear. When disk degeneration is advanced (for example, loss of intervertebral height, osteophyte formation, facet hypertrophy), the patient may also exhibit signs and symptoms of spinal stenosis and/or radiculopathy.

Untreated AIS may or may not progress into adulthood, and symptoms may or may not develop over time. Weinstein et al[21] followed 161 patients and found that back pain, the most common symptom at long-term follow-up, was present in 37% of patients at a mean age of 39.3 years. Interestingly, the incidence of back pain did not correlate with the severity of the curve, but it was higher (52%) in patients with thoracolumbar curves. Restricted pulmonary function may develop as a consequence of untreated AIS. Restricted pulmonary function was most commonly associated with thoracic curves (41% at long-term follow-up) and correlated with the severity of the curve.[21] Neurologic symptoms may develop in adult patients as a result of curve progression and degenerative changes, and these patients may have symptoms related to neurogenic claudication, myelopathy, or radiculopathy. Patients with a sagittal imbalance of the spine may experience muscle fatigue after prolonged standing or walking.

Evaluation
Physical Examination
Physical examination involves observation of gait, with particular attention paid to the patient's sagittal and coronal spinal alignment, the presence of a forward-flexed posture during ambulation, and weakness in dorsiflexion or plantar flexion of the ankles. Spinal mobility in flexion and extension with associated pain observed during these maneuvers should be carefully documented. Flexion may be limited in the presence of advanced spondylolisthesis, paraspinal muscle spasm, or severe hamstring contracture. A midline step-off of the spinous processes of L5 and S1 may be detected during palpation in spondylolisthesis. A full neurologic examination is indicated to detect weakness, sensory loss, or abnormal deep tendon reflexes. The entire back should be visible to examine for compensatory hyperlordosis, which is often noted above the level of a slip in advanced spondylolisthesis. The physical examination of the patient with scoliosis should include evaluation for limb-length discrepancy, symmetry of shoulder heights, degrees of lumbar lordosis and thoracic kyphosis, rib prominence, and truncopelvic balance. The Adams forward bend test is sensitive for detecting even mild degrees of asymmetry of the ribcage and the low back.

Imaging Studies
Weight-bearing AP, lateral, and oblique radiographs of the lumbosacral spine are required to evaluate for spondylolisthesis. A pars defect, if present, can be seen on a collimated lateral view of the lumbosacral spine 84% of the time[28] (**Figure 1**), and in an additional 5% of patients who actually have a defect, it can be observed on an oblique view. If radiographs are inconclusive and spondylolysis is suspected, a CT scan provides the greatest detail of the pars interarticularis and can identify a defect that may not appear on routine radiographs. If the chronicity of the defect is in question, a single-photon emission CT scan can be obtained; however, active isthmic lesions in adults are rare (**Figure 2**).

The adult patients who had AIS are evaluated using full-length weight-bearing AP, lateral, and side-bending radiographs. CT and MRI provide additional bony and soft-tissue delineation, respectively, for diagnostic and preoperative planning purposes.

FIGURE 1

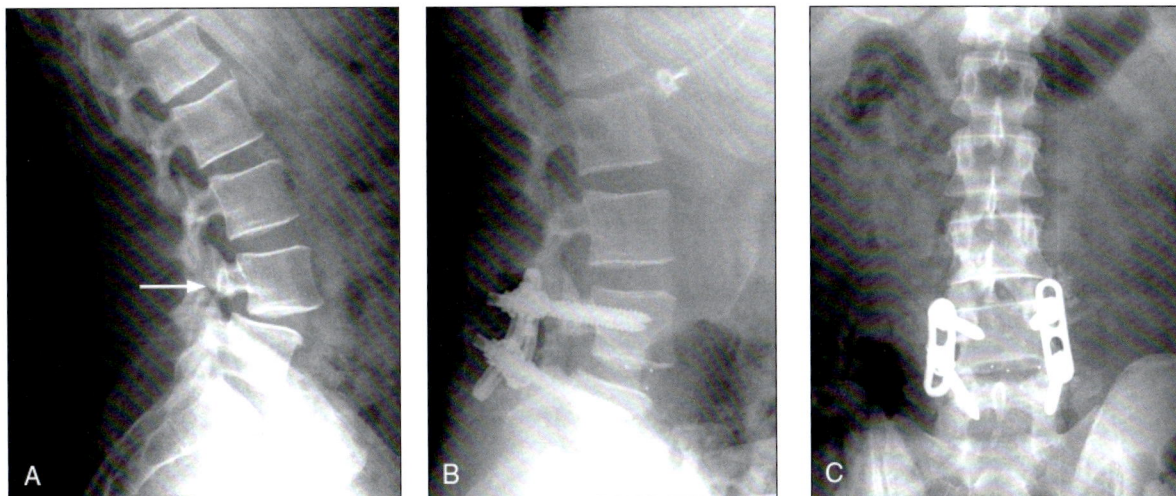

Radiographs of a 44-year-old man who presented with disabling low back pain despite nonsurgical treatment. **A,** Preoperative lateral view shows a bilateral isthmic defect (arrow). Postoperative lateral (**B**) and AP (**C**) views show an L4-L5 transforaminal lumbar interbody fusion and posterolateral fusion.

INTERVENTIONS FOR THE ADULT PATIENT
Literature Review

A long-term follow-up study by Beutler et al[17] suggested an overall benign course of isthmic spondylolisthesis into adulthood. As such, patients in whom spondylolysis and spondylolisthesis was diagnosed in childhood can be expected to have a clinical course similar to that of the general population. The degree of slip in childhood directly correlates with the degree of degeneration of the L5-S1 intervertebral disk in adulthood. Patients with spondylolysis and spondylolisthesis have been found to have greater radiographic evidence of L5-S1 disk degeneration when compared with asymptomatic adult control groups.[17,29,30] As patients with isthmic spondylolisthesis age (for example, at follow-up at age 45 years or older), they may develop back pain more often than patients in age-matched control groups.[17] As with all adult patients with back pain, those with spondylolisthesis and/or spondylolysis will require a comprehensive evaluation to determine the etiology of pain because the presence of spondylolysis or spondylolisthesis may be incidental and may delay the diagnosis and appropriate intervention for other causes of low back pain.

In a 2-year follow-up study by Fritzell et al,[31] patients with debilitating chronic low back pain and radiographic evidence of disk degeneration were randomized into either surgical or nonsurgical treatment groups. At final follow-up, only 63% of surgical patients thought that their back pain improved with surgery. Additional randomized studies have failed to show the superiority of surgical over nonsurgical treatment in patients with chronic low back pain.[32,33] With these data in mind, adult patients with a history of spondylolysis or spondylolisthesis should be treated similarly to any other adult patient with back pain. The literature suggests that nonsurgical care is most effective.

In 1981, Weinstein et al[21] found that back pain occurs more frequently in adult patients who had AIS when compared with control patients and is the most common indication for surgical intervention in adulthood. Takahashi et al[34] conducted a surgical outcomes study of adult patients in whom AIS was previously diagnosed. The authors found that pain was present in 95% of patients older than 40 years. In a similar outcomes study in 2003 by Ali et al,[35] back pain was the indication for surgery (with or without deformity progression) in 83% of patients. Although nonsurgical care should always

FIGURE 2

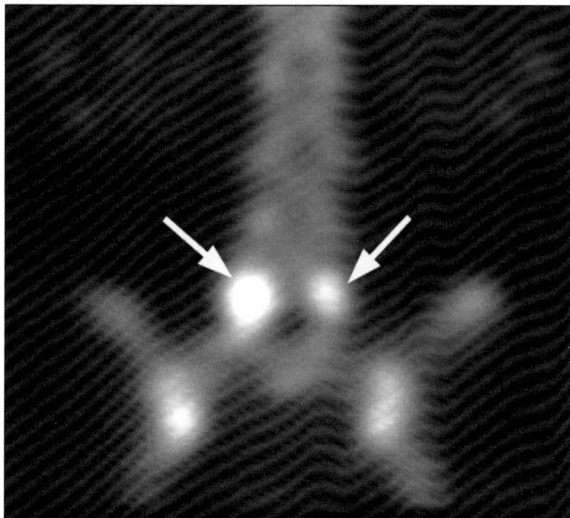

Single-photon emission CT scan shows increased uptake at the right and left regions of the pars interarticularis of L5 (arrows) in a 13-year-old boy with back pain.

be the initial treatment plan, intractable and persistent back pain is an indication for surgical intervention.

Nonsurgical Treatment

Adults with spondylolysis and isthmic spondylolisthesis who are asymptomatic do not require treatment, and may be followed up on an as-needed basis. Many individuals with spondylolytic lesions remain asymptomatic during their lifetimes, so when symptoms develop in these patients, a thorough search for other sources of pain should be conducted. When more ominous lesions are ruled out, these patients are treated as would any other adult patient with low back pain. In the acute setting, the patient is instructed to remain active within his or her pain limits. Bed rest has been recommended for acute pain exacerbations; however, evidence does not support this treatment.[36] Physical therapy and NSAIDs also may be used, and narcotic drugs should be avoided. If symptoms persist for 4 to 6 weeks, MRI evaluation may help detect neural compression and may provide information regarding the status of the intervertebral disks. Diskography may be helpful when the etiology of back pain is unclear or when multiple levels of disk degeneration are present. When intolerable back pain

and/or leg pain remain unresolved after nonsurgical treatment, surgical intervention may be indicated.

Back pain that develops in adult patients with AIS is generally treated nonsurgically. In the presence of coexisting spinal stenosis, epidural steroid injections and selective nerve root blocks are important components of the treatment plan. Physical therapy programs should emphasize core muscle strengthening and stretching of the low back. Core muscle strengthening programs impart additional stability to the unstable segments and may ultimately reduce pain. Patients with unremitting back pain and/or leg pain in whom nonsurgical treatment has failed are candidates for surgical intervention; however, this option should be considered only after the patient has a thorough understanding of the risks of surgery, which are significant in this patient population.

Surgical Treatment

Various surgical treatment options exist for the adult patient with symptomatic spondylolysis or spondylolisthesis. Direct repair of the pars defect is an acceptable treatment option for children, but this option is not recommended in the adult population with secondary degenerative changes. In the adult, surgical interventions include fusion (with or without decompression) of the posterolateral elements (PLF), anterior lumbar interbody fusion (ALIF), transforaminal lumbar interbody fusion (TLIF), posterior lumbar interbody fusion (PLIF), and interbody fusion supplemented with posterior fixation (with or without PLF). Posterior techniques allow direct decompression of the neural elements, deformity correction, and rigid stabilization. PLF is a technique familiar to spine surgeons and does not require an access surgeon; however, clinical and radiographic success rates in adult patients treated with PLF are inferior to those treated with an interbody fusion procedure.[37-42] The clinical success rates of decompression and PLF are inferior to those for PLF alone because of a presumed increase in instability created by decompression.[43,44] These clinical observations serve as the basis for the recommendation of interbody fusion for isthmic spondylolisthesis in adults.

ALIF procedures do not allow direct decompression of the neural elements; however, indirect decompression of the neuroforamina and partial reduction of the slip may be achieved by increasing the intervertebral height

FIGURE 3

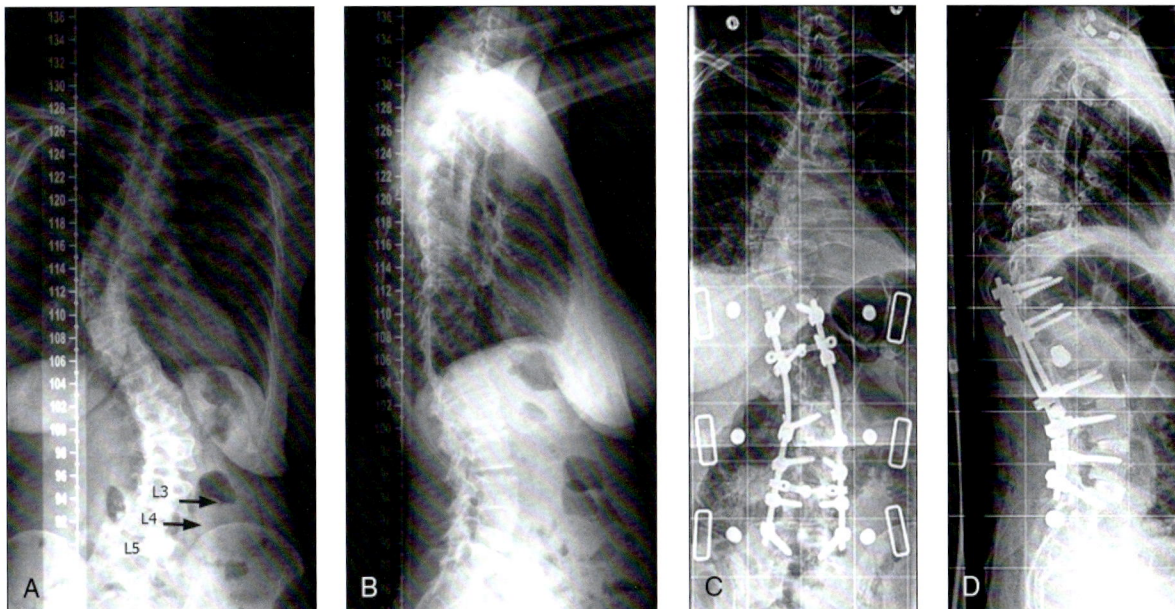

Radiographs of a 45-year-old woman who presented with bilateral radiculopathy and low back pain unrelieved by nonsurgical treatment. Preoperative AP (**A**) and lateral (**B**) views show the L3-L4 and L4-L5 lateral listhesis (arrows, **A**) and collapse, which corresponded to the patient's radicular symptoms. Postoperative AP (**C**) and lateral (**D**) views show anterior lumbar interbody fusion of L2-L3 through L4-L5 anterior lumbar interbody fusion using structural allografts, followed by an L3-L5 laminectomy and a T11-L5 posterior fusion and instrumentation using iliac crest autograft and local bone.

using interbody graft placement. ALIF procedures allow a more thorough diskectomy and end plate preparation when compared with the more limited interspace access provided by the PLIF or TLIF procedure. Patients treated using ALIF experience less pain than those treated with posterior approaches. Despite the advantages of ALIF, the process is associated with significant risks. In male patients, disruption of the sympathetic plexus can cause retrograde ejaculation. In addition, the risk of catastrophic vessel injury and damage to retroperitoneal and intraperitoneal structures exists in all patients treated with anterior surgery.

Although adult patients with isthmic spondylolisthesis undergoing stand-alone ALIFs appear to do well at long-term follow-up,[45-47] ALIFs are often combined with posterior instrumentation with or without PLF. The highest fusion rates in adult patients are reported with combined interbody and posterolateral fusion, also known as circumferential fusion.[48,49] For combined anterior and posterior approaches, many studies that report higher fusion rates with circumferential fusion procedures (versus PLF alone) fail to show significant improvements in clinical outcomes.[39,48,49]

Back pain may occur in the adult patient with AIS and is a common reason for surgical intervention. The principles of surgical treatment include correction of sagittal and coronal spinal imbalance, direct decompression of stenosis that is unlikely to improve with indirect decompression alone, and the inclusion of spinal segments thought to be contributing to back pain, when possible (**Figure 3**). In addition, the caudal vertebra of a fusion construct should not be in a kyphotic segment and should be flexible enough to be brought into neutral position in a sidebending radiograph. These goals are generally accomplished via a posterior approach, but an anterior release and interbody fusion may be required in rigid segments that prohibit restoration of sagittal and coronal plane alignment. Using contemporary pedicle screw fixation techniques, Ali et al[35] reported on minimum 2-year follow-up of surgically treated adult patients with idiopathic scoliosis. The authors noted that 65% of patients were no longer taking pain medication, 70% of patients were able to exercise and perform recreational activities, and 95% of patients would choose to undergo the same treatment again.

EXPERT OPINION
Evaluation

To alert the physician to more ominous conditions than those described in this chapter, a thorough history and physical examination should be conducted for any patient with unremitting back pain. Advanced imaging should be undertaken when indicated.

For patients with spondylolysis or isthmic spondylolisthesis, the history should be directed at characterizing the nature of the pain in the hopes of most accurately defining its etiology. For example, pain that is worse while sitting versus when standing suggests diskogenic pain, whereas pain that is worse while standing suggests pain from arthrosis of the facet joints. The examination should focus on detecting neurologic deficits. Imaging studies should include AP, lateral, and flexion-extension radiographs of the lumbosacral spine. An oblique radiograph may demonstrate a pars defect that is not evident on routine images. A CT scan of the lumbosacral spine more accurately defines any pars defect and facet hypertrophy. CT also documents pedicle size and trajectory in anticipation of pedicle screw fixation. MRI allows accurate assessment of the central canal, the lateral recesses, and the foramina, as well as the hydration status of the intervertebral disks. Diskography may provide useful information in determining or confirming the responsible intervertebral segment in suspected diskogenic back pain.

Adult patients with AIS and back pain should be evaluated in a similar manner. The possibility of a more ominous diagnosis should be investigated if indicated by the history and physical examination. Once other causes of pain are ruled out, imaging of the spine should include full-length weight-bearing AP and lateral radiographs of the thoracic and lumbar spine. On the weight-bearing AP view, the C7 plumb line should be within 2 cm of the center of the sacrum. On the lateral view, the C7 plumb line should be within 4 cm of the posterior lumbosacral disk. Flexion-extension and sidebending radiographs can elucidate instability that may be present and may provide useful information concerning the rigidity of the curves. CT and MRI can provide additional information that is helpful for both diagnostic and preoperative planning purposes.

Preferred Interventions

For symptomatic adult patients with spondylolysis and spondylolisthesis in whom nonsurgical treatment has failed, we favor circumferential fusion procedures. To achieve this goal for a low-grade minimally kyphotic (or lordotic) interspace, we prefer to perform a TLIF procedure. However, the specific procedure of choice should take into account the surgeon's experience, the availability and skill of an access surgeon (if an anterior approach is considered), and the patient's preference. Each approach has inherent risks and benefits, and the final decision should be made only after the patient has a full understanding of each approach.

In the adult patient with idiopathic scoliosis in whom extensive nonsurgical treatment (at least 6 to 12 weeks) has failed, surgery may be warranted. These patients are often elderly, have multiple comorbid conditions, and are at significant risk for complications. Achieving proper sagittal and coronal spinal balance is extremely important and takes precedence over fixing a curve. Patients with a residual imbalance (for example, with a C7 plumb line 10 cm anterior to the lumbosacral disk) will have poor results.[50]

The fusion construct should not end at a tilted lumbar segment; at a degenerated, painful, or arthritic segment; or in a kyphotic region. We believe the lumbosacral disk should be included in the fusion construct in the presence of segmental instability, when coexistent stenosis requires decompression at the lumbosacral level, when there is a fixed obliquity of the lumbosacral motion segment, when advanced degenerative changes are present at L5-S1, and when sagittal and/or coronal balance cannot otherwise be obtained.

The necessity of a combined anterior/posterior approach versus a posterior-only approach is dictated by the severity and rigidity of the curve. As a general rule, we have found that thoracic curves less than 70° and thoracolumbar and lumbar curves less than 60° can be successfully treated using a posterior approach. Severely scoliotic curves may require anterior release and inter-body fusion, either with a staged procedure or on the same day. In addition, a combined anterior/posterior approach should be considered in patients with significant lumbar kyphosis (>30°), when extension to the sacrum is anticipated, and when significant osteoporosis is present. An alternative approach to the patient with significant lumbar kyphosis is a pedicle subtraction osteotomy, but this procedure is associated with increased blood loss and morbidity and is more technically demanding. The surgeon's experience and the availability and skill of an access surgeon are the most important factors in determining how restoration of lumbar lordosis is achieved.

CONCLUSION

Spondylolysis, spondylolisthesis, and scoliosis are commonly seen in both children and adults. As with all spinal conditions, proper diagnosis and treatment begins with a thorough history, physical examination, and appropriate imaging studies. These conditions are often asymptomatic; therefore, conditions unrelated to the spine when evaluating back or leg pain should be considered. Initial treatment should always be nonsurgical when the conditions are symptomatic. Surgical treatment may be indicated if nonsurgical measures fail. Often, many surgical options exist, and after an informed discussion with the patient, the approach chosen should consider the nature of the pathology and the surgeon's experience.

REFERENCES

1. Wiltse LL, Newman PH, Macnab I: Classification of spondylolisis and spondylolisthesis. *Clin Orthop Relat Res* 1976(117):23-29.
2. Fredrickson BE, Baker D, McHolick WJ, Yuan HA, Lubicky JP: The natural history of spondylolysis and spondylolisthesis. *J Bone Joint Surg Am* 1984;66(5):699-707.
3. Simper LB: Spondylolysis in Eskimo skeletons. *Acta Orthop Scand* 1986;57(1):78-80.
4. Rowe GG, Roche MB: The etiology of separate neural arch. *J Bone Joint Surg Am* 1953;35-A(1):102-110.
5. Albanese M, Pizzutillo PD: Family study of spondylolysis and spondylolisthesis. *J Pediatr Orthop* 1982;2(5):496-499.
6. Micheli LJ, Wood R: Back pain in young athletes: Significant differences from adults in causes and patterns. *Arch Pediatr Adolesc Med* 1995;149(1):15-18.
7. Congeni J, McCulloch J, Swanson K: Lumbar spondylolysis: A study of natural progression in athletes. *Am J Sports Med* 1997;25(2):248-253.
8. Rosenberg NJ, Bargar WL, Friedman B: The incidence of spondylolysis and spondylolisthesis in nonambulatory patients. *Spine (Phila Pa 1976)* 1981;6(1):35-38.
9. Shands AR Jr, Eisberg HB: The incidence of scoliosis in the state of Delaware; a study of 50,000 minifilms of the chest made during a survey for tuberculosis. *J Bone Joint Surg Am* 1955;37-A(6):1243-1249.
10. Lonstein JE, Bjorklund S, Wanninger MH, Nelson RP: Voluntary school screening for scoliosis in Minnesota. *J Bone Joint Surg Am* 1982;64(4):481-488.
11. Carr AJ: Adolescent idiopathic scoliosis in identical twins. *J Bone Joint Surg Br* 1990;72(6):1077.
12. Harrington PR: The etiology of idiopathic scoliosis. *Clin Orthop Relat Res* 1977(126):17-25.
13. Gurnett CA, Alaee F, Bowcock A, et al: Genetic linkage localizes an adolescent idiopathic scoliosis and pectus excavatum gene to chromosome 18 q. *Spine (Phila Pa 1976)* 2009;34(2):E94-E100.
14. Zhang HQ, Lu SJ, Tang MX, et al: Association of estrogen receptor beta gene polymorphisms with susceptibility to adolescent idiopathic scoliosis. *Spine (Phila Pa 1976)* 2009;34(8):760-764.
15. Wise CA, Gao X, Shoemaker S, Gordon D, Herring JA: Understanding genetic factors in idiopathic scoliosis, a complex disease of childhood. *Curr Genomics* 2008;9(1):51-59.
16. Weinstein SL: Idiopathic scoliosis: Natural history. *Spine (Phila Pa 1976)* 1986;11(8):780-783.
17. Beutler WJ, Fredrickson BE, Murtland A, Sweeney CA, Grant WD, Baker D: The natural history of spondylolysis and spondylolisthesis: 45-year follow-up evaluation. *Spine (Phila Pa 1976)* 2003;28(10):1027-1035.
18. Saraste H: Long-term clinical and radiological follow-up of spondylolysis and spondylolisthesis. *J Pediatr Orthop* 1987;7(6):631-638.
19. Lonstein JE, Carlson JM: The prediction of curve progression in untreated idiopathic scoliosis during growth. *J Bone Joint Surg Am* 1984;66(7):1061-1071.
20. Weinstein SL, Ponseti IV: Curve progression in idiopathic scoliosis. *J Bone Joint Surg Am* 1983;65(4):447-455.

21. Weinstein SL, Zavala DC, Ponseti IV: Idiopathic scoliosis: Long-term follow-up and prognosis in untreated patients. *J Bone Joint Surg Am* 1981;63(5):702-712.

22. Pizzutillo PD, Hummer CD III: Nonoperative treatment for painful adolescent spondylolysis or spondylolisthesis. *J Pediatr Orthop* 1989;9(5):538-540.

23. Klein G, Mehlman CT, McCarty M: Nonoperative treatment of spondylolysis and grade I spondylolisthesis in children and young adults: A meta-analysis of observational studies. *J Pediatr Orthop* 2009;29(2):146-156.

24. Fujii K, Katoh S, Sairyo K, Ikata T, Yasui N: Union of defects in the pars interarticularis of the lumbar spine in children and adolescents: The radiological outcome after conservative treatment. *J Bone Joint Surg Br* 2004;86(2):225-231.

25. Lamberg TS, Remes VM, Helenius IJ, et al: Long-term clinical, functional and radiological outcome 21 years after posterior or posterolateral fusion in childhood and adolescence isthmic spondylolisthesis. *Eur Spine J* 2005;14(7):639-644.

26. Molinari RW, Bridwell KH, Lenke LG, Ungacta FF, Riew KD: Complications in the surgical treatment of pediatric high-grade, isthmic dysplastic spondylolisthesis: A comparison of three surgical approaches. *Spine (Phila Pa 1976)* 1999;24(16):1701-1711.

27. Lehman RA Jr, Lenke LG, Keeler KA, et al: Operative treatment of adolescent idiopathic scoliosis with posterior pedicle screw-only constructs: Minimum three-year follow-up of one hundred fourteen cases. *Spine (Phila Pa 1976)* 2008;33(14):1598-1604.

28. Amato M, Totty WG, Gilula LA: Spondylolysis of the lumbar spine: Demonstration of defects and laminal fragmentation. *Radiology* 1984;153(3):627-629.

29. Boden SD, Davis DO, Dina TS, Patronas NJ, Wiesel SW: Abnormal magnetic-resonance scans of the lumbar spine in asymptomatic subjects: A prospective investigation. *J Bone Joint Surg Am* 1990;72(3):403-408.

30. Jarvik JJ, Hollingworth W, Heagerty P, Haynor DR, Deyo RA: The Longitudinal Assessment of Imaging and Disability of the Back (LAIDBack) Study: Baseline data. *Spine (Phila Pa 1976)* 2001;26(10):1158-1166.

31. Fritzell P, Hägg O, Wessberg P, Nordwall A; Swedish Lumbar Spine Study Group: 2001 Volvo Award Winner in Clinical Studies: Lumbar fusion versus nonsurgical treatment for chronic low back pain. A multicenter randomized controlled trial from the Swedish Lumbar Spine Study Group. *Spine (Phila Pa 1976)* 2001;26(23):2521-2534.

32. Brox JI, Sørensen R, Friis A, et al: Randomized clinical trial of lumbar instrumented fusion and cognitive intervention and exercises in patients with chronic low back pain and disc degeneration. *Spine (Phila Pa 1976)* 2003;28(17):1913-1921.

33. Fairbank J, Frost H, Wilson-MacDonald J, et al: Randomised controlled trial to compare surgical stabilisation of the lumbar spine with an intensive rehabilitation programme for patients with chronic low back pain: The MRC spine stabilisation trial. *BMJ* 2005;330(7502):1233.

34. Takahashi S, Delécrin J, Passuti N: Surgical treatment of idiopathic scoliosis in adults: An age-related analysis of outcome. *Spine (Phila Pa 1976)* 2002;27(16):1742-1748.

35. Ali RM, Boachie-Adjei O, Rawlins BA: Functional and radiographic outcomes after surgery for adult scoliosis using third-generation instrumentation techniques. *Spine (Phila Pa 1976)* 2003;28(11):1163-1170.

36. Hilde G, Hagen KB, Jamtvedt G, Winnem M: Advice to stay active as a single treatment for low back pain and sciatica. *Cochrane Database Syst Rev* 2002;2(2):CD003632.

37. Barrick WT, Schofferman JA, Reynolds JB, et al: Anterior lumbar fusion improves discogenic pain at levels of prior posterolateral fusion. *Spine (Phila Pa 1976)* 2000;25(7):853-857.

38. L'Heureux EA Jr, Perra JH, Pinto MR, Smith MD, Denis F, Lonstein JE: Functional outcome analysis including preoperative and postoperative SF-36 for surgically treated adult isthmic spondylolisthesis. *Spine (Phila Pa 1976)* 2003;28(12):1269-1274.

39. La Rosa G, Conti A, Cacciola F, et al: Pedicle screw fixation for isthmic spondylolisthesis: Does posterior lumbar interbody fusion improve outcome over posterolateral fusion? *J Neurosurg* 2003;99(Suppl 2)143-150.

40. Johnsson R, Strömqvist B, Axelsson P, Selvik G: Influence of spinal immobilization on consolidation of posterolateral lumbosacral fusion: A roentgen stereophotogrammetric and radiographic analysis. *Spine (Phila Pa 1976)* 1992;17(1):16-21.

41. Lenke LG, Bridwell KH, Bullis D, Betz RR, Baldus C, Schoenecker PL: Results of in situ fusion for isthmic spondylolisthesis. *J Spinal Disord* 1992;5(4):433-442.

42. Vaccaro AR, Ring D, Scuderi G, Cohen DS, Garfin SR: Predictors of outcome in patients with chronic back pain and low-grade spondylolisthesis. *Spine (Phila Pa 1976)* 1997;22(17):2030-2035.

43. Carragee EJ: Single-level posterolateral arthrodesis, with or without posterior decompression, for the treatment of isthmic spondylolisthesis in adults: A prospective, randomized study. *J Bone Joint Surg Am* 1997;79(8):1175-1180.

44. de Loubresse CG, Bon T, Deburge A, Lassale B, Benoit M: Posterolateral fusion for radicular pain in isthmic spondylolisthesis. *Clin Orthop Relat Res* 1996(323): 194-201.

45. Cheng CL, Fang D, Lee PC, Leong JC: Anterior spinal fusion for spondylolysis and isthmic spondylolisthesis: Long term results in adults. *J Bone Joint Surg Br* 1989;71(2):264-267.

46. Ishihara H, Osada R, Kanamori M, et al: Minimum 10-year follow-up study of anterior lumbar interbody fusion for isthmic spondylolisthesis. *J Spinal Disord* 2001;14(2):91-99.

47. van Rens TJ, van Horn JR: Long-term results in lumbosacral interbody fusion for spondylolisthesis. *Acta Orthop Scand* 1982;53(3):383-392.

48. Suk SI, Lee CK, Kim WJ, Lee JH, Cho KJ, Kim HG: Adding posterior lumbar interbody fusion to pedicle screw fixation and posterolateral fusion after decompression in spondylolytic spondylolisthesis. *Spine (Phila Pa 1976)* 1997;22(2):210-220.

49. Madan S, Boeree NR: Outcome of posterior lumbar interbody fusion versus posterolateral fusion for spondylolytic spondylolisthesis. *Spine (Phila Pa 1976)* 2002;27(14):1536-1542.

50. Glassman SD, Bridwell K, Dimar JR, Horton W, Berven S, Schwab F: The impact of positive sagittal balance in adult spinal deformity. *Spine (Phila Pa 1976)* 2005;30(18):2024-2029.

HIP DISORDERS: DEVELOPMENTAL DYSPLASIA, SLIPPED CAPITAL FEMORAL EPIPHYSIS, AND LEGG-CALVÉ-PERTHES DISEASE

MICHAEL B. MILLIS, MD
EDUARDO N. NOVAIS, MD

INTRODUCTION

Pediatric and adolescent hip disorders, including developmental dysplasia of the hip (DDH), slipped capital femoral epiphysis (SCFE), and Legg-Calvé-Perthes (LCP) disease, may be asymptomatic during adolescence and early adulthood. However, these conditions may be associated with structural deformities of the proximal femur and the acetabulum that create a destructive mechanical environment for the hip. Mechanical dysfunction of the hip has been recognized as a major factor in the etiology of osteoarthritis of the hip joint.[1,2] Symptomatic osteoarthritis of the hip is the major adult consequence of these pediatric and adolescent hip conditions.[3-7]

Osteoarthritis of the hip has been categorized as primary (also called idiopathic, meaning unclear cause; suspected primary undetermined abnormality of the cartilage or the subchondral bone) or secondary (caused by recognized structural abnormalities that often are congenital or developmental). In the 1950s, approximately 60% of end-stage hip osteoarthritis cases were believed to be primary.[8] In 1965, Murray[5] described the tilt deformity of the proximal femur as a possible cause of osteoarthritis. In the 1970s, Stulberg and Harris[9] examined the radiographs of 75 patients with idiopathic osteoarthritis of the hip and found that 39% had acetabular dysplasia, as determined by using four measurements of acetabular configuration. An additional 40% of the patients were found to have a pistol grip deformity of the proximal femur.[7] Solomon[6,10] and Harris[11] clearly demonstrated that most cases of hip osteoarthritis previously thought to be primary are associated with a developmental hip deformity that may not have been recognized before skeletal maturity. In 1986, Aronson[3] reported that 76% of hips that underwent total hip arthroplasty had associated diagnoses of pediatric hip disease (43% DDH, 22% SCFE, and 11% LCP disease).

ETIOLOGY OF HIP DISORDERS

Ganz et al[12] first recognized and described femoroacetabular impingement (FAI) as a major etiologic factor in many cases of hip osteoarthritis for which the development was previously not understood. FAI has been described as an abnormal and mechanically problem-

Neither of the following authors nor any immediate family member has received anything of value from or has stock or stock options held in a commercial company or institution related directly or indirectly to the subject of this chapter: Dr. Millis and Dr. Novais.

atic contact between the proximal femur and the anterior aspect of the acetabular rim. FAI has been linked to early-onset hip osteoarthritis.[12-14] FAI is currently divided into two major categories: cam type (deformities of the femoral head-neck junction) and pincer type (acetabular overcoverage of the femoral head).[12] FAI has been recognized as the mechanism of articular damage not only in symptomatic patients following SCFE and LCP disease, but also in patients without previously recognized hip disease[2] in whom the problem appears to have a developmental basis.[15] Cam-type FAI was seen on MRI in 24% of young asymptomatic males and in 48% of males with internal rotation of the hip less than 30°.[16]

A Mechanical Paradigm for Osteoarthritis of the Hip

Models for normal and abnormal hip mechanics have been described by Pauwels[17] and Bombelli.[1,18] Abnormal mechanics, often associated with instability, impingement, or a combination of both, may ultimately result in osteoarthritis of the hip joint.[2] Early clinical manifestations of mechanical hip problems often originate at the acetabular rim. This is called acetabular rim syndrome and was first described by Klaue et al.[19] Patients with acetabular rim syndrome may present with hip impingement as well as rim damage secondary to instability from dysplasia or a combination of instability and FAI.

Hip-Preserving Techniques for the Mature Hip

Contemporary hip-preserving surgical techniques should be justified as improving or correcting an identified mechanical abnormality that is causing symptoms or may compromise hip function.[20] These techniques correct abnormalities before structural damage to articular cartilage has occurred. Established articular damage is the primary obstacle to achieving excellent results in hip-preserving surgery. Because articular damage is cumulative, early diagnosis of mechanical abnormality is extremely important in hip preservation. Useful hip-preserving techniques in the mature hip at risk for mechanical failure include periacetabular realignment osteotomies (open approaches); proximal femur realignment osteotomies (open approaches); osteo-

chondroplasty of the acetabulum and/or the femoral head-neck junction (open, arthroscopic, or combined approaches); and direct surgery performed on the labrum or articular cartilage (open, arthroscopic, or combined approaches).

DEVELOPMENTAL DYSPLASIA OF THE HIP
Incidence

The true incidence of DDH is difficult to establish because of its wide spectrum of severity, ranging from acetabular dysplasia to subluxated and dislocated hips, as well as wide variations that occur among ethnic groups.[21] Although more than 60% of infants with DDH have no identifiable risk factor, having both a first-degree relative with DDH and a breech delivery are high risk factors.[22] The incidence of DDH with clinical and ultrasonographic screening is 5.0 cases per 1,000 live births.[23] DDH is also discussed in detail in chapter 3.

Common Childhood Interventions and Outcomes

The goal of treating DDH in childhood is to obtain and maintain concentric reduction of the hip to stimulate the acetabulum to resume normal development.[24] Children of walking age usually are best treated with open reduction. Schoenecker et al[25] reported that the chance of obtaining a closed reduction in infants older than 18 months is 70%, and two thirds of patients require secondary procedures after closed reduction of the hip.[26,27] Open reduction of the hip may be performed through a medial[28] or an anteromedial[29-31] approach in children up to 2 years of age; however, residual acetabular dysplasia is common and secondary procedures are necessary in 25% to 50% of these hips.[30,32] The anterolateral approach, often combined with a femoral shortening osteotomy, is the most accepted method for open reduction in a child older than 2 years.[33]

Albinana et al[34] reported that an acetabular index of 35° or more at 2-year follow-up after reduction was associated with an 80% probability of a poor outcome. The older the child with residual dysplasia, the more likely that realignment osteotomy of the proximal femur,[35] pelvis,[36,37] or both[38] will be required for optimal function both in childhood and adulthood. A long-

FIGURE 1

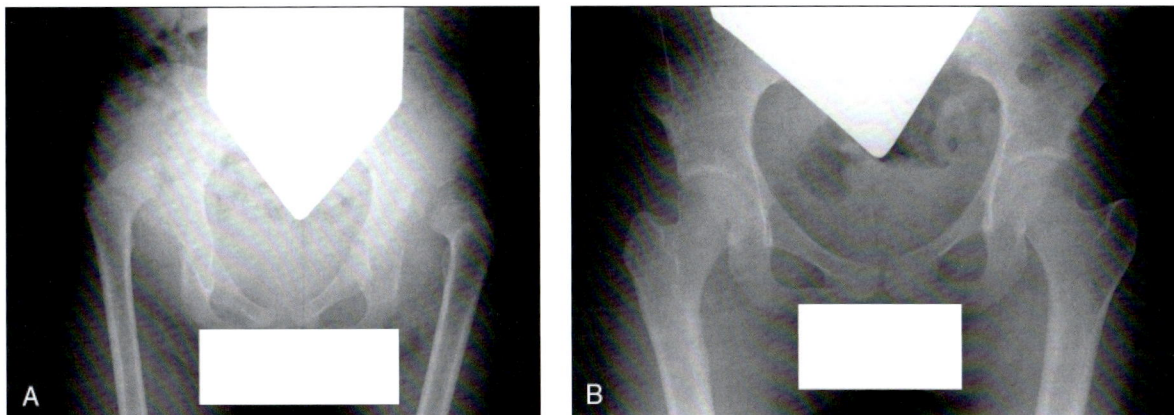

Radiographs of the pelvis in a girl born with bilateral developmental dysplasia of the hip. The dislocation in both hips is high and severe. **A,** AP view obtained at 5 years of age reveals the high-riding femoral heads and the false acetabulum. **B,** AP view obtained at 15 years of age reveals bilateral concentric reduction with normal femoral head coverage, with no signs of arthritis.

term study that followed patients who presented after 18 months of age and who underwent open reduction of the hip and pelvic Salter osteotomy reported a failure rate (requiring total hip arthroplasty) of 46% of the surviving hips and definite osteoarthritis in 25%.[39,40] In general, unilateral DDH represents an indication for surgical treatment because of the association of secondary spinal problems, hyperlordosis, and ipsilateral limb shortening. Bilateral DDH diagnosed after walking age may be treated surgically in children up to 6 years of age (**Figure 1**). In children older than 6 years, not only is there the risk of a stiff, painful hip on at least one side as the result of a primary bilateral open reduction, but leaving the hips unreduced gives a functional and pain-free result for decades. The prognosis for untreated complete dislocation of the hip depends on two factors: bilaterality and the presence of a false acetabulum.[41]

Residual acetabular dysplasia in the reduced hip is most commonly treated using a realignment pelvic osteotomy, such as the incomplete Pemberton osteotomy,[37] Dega osteotomy,[42,43] or complete Salter innominate osteotomy.[36] One concern with the complete Salter innominate osteotomy is retroversion of the acetabular dome, which could lead to FAI in adulthood[44] (**Figure 2**). In older children with severe dysplasia, triple pelvic osteotomy may be indicated before closure of the triradiate cartilage.

Adult Sequelae

After closure of triradiate cartilage, issues involving the dysplastic hip in the adolescent are similar to those in the adult that are known to lead to secondary osteoarthritis.[9,11] Murphy et al[45] noted no patient had a well-functioning hip at age 65 years if the lateral center-edge angle was less than 16°, the acetabular index of depth to width was less than 38%, the acetabular index of the weight-bearing zone was greater than 15°, the uncovering of the femoral head was greater than 31%, or the peak-to-edge distance was 0. Hip subluxation is a major risk factor for the development of early arthritis[46]

Presenting Symptoms

The skeletally mature patient with hip dysplasia frequently presents with no history of hip disorders. The initial problem, usually unnoticed for months or years by the patient, is a mild activity-related limp, accompanied by a mild ache over the greater trochanter or lateral thigh. As the labrum and the anterior acetabular rim become injured, groin pain begins.[19] Symptoms of locking, catching, and/or instability develop as rim damage increases.

Evaluation

A pertinent clinical interview should include a family history, birth history, and childhood history, especially

FIGURE 2

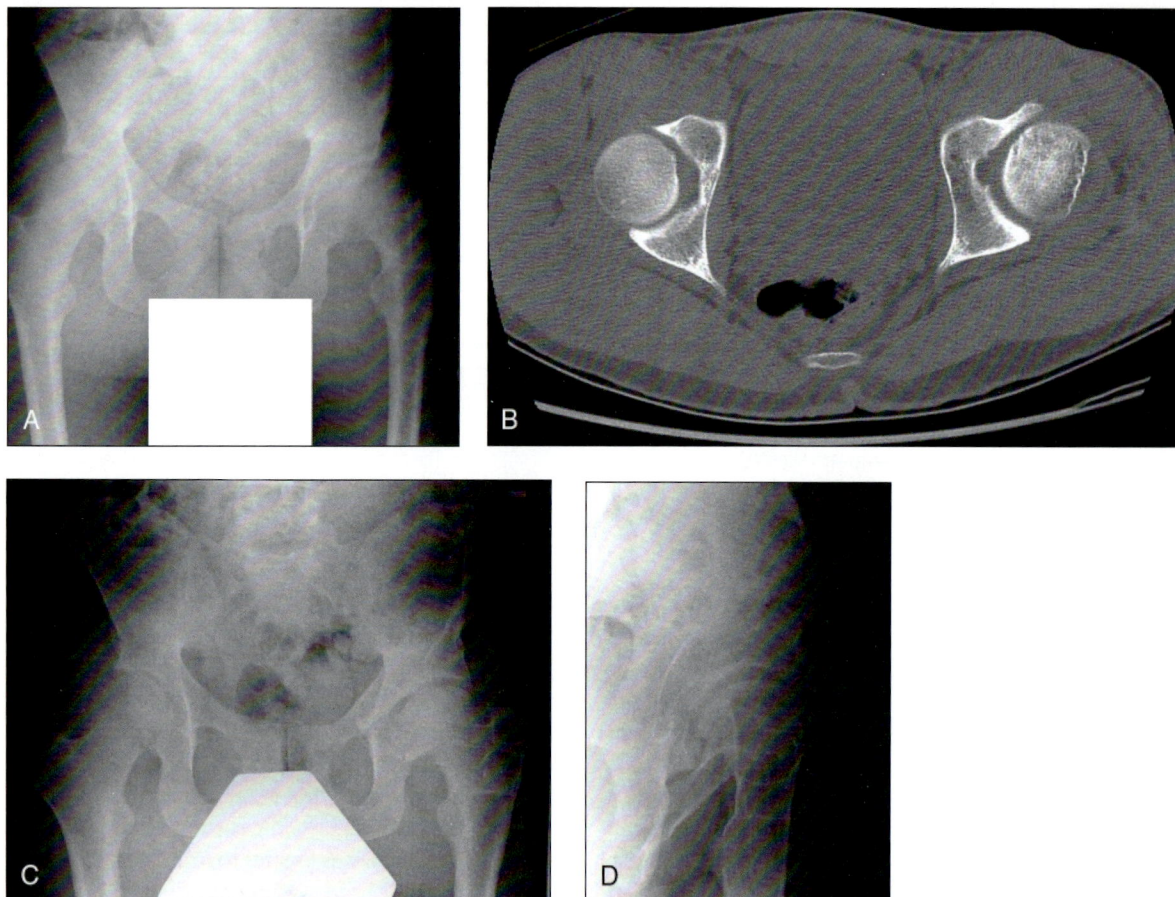

Imaging studies of the pelvis of an 18-year-old man who underwent a Salter osteotomy, open reduction, and femoral osteotomy as a child. **A,** AP radiograph shows reduced coverage of the femoral head laterally and retroversion of the left acetabulum (a positive crossover sign). **B,** Axial CT scan better shows acetabular retroversion. AP (**C**) and false-profile (**D**) views obtained at 5-year follow-up demonstrate appropriate correction, with restored acetabular version and improved coverage of the femoral head.

involving general orthopaedic and hip conditions. Neuromuscular conditions such as Charcot-Marie-Tooth disease should be ruled out in a patient who presents later in life with hip dysplasia. Detailed characterization of any existing hip symptoms should include date of onset, location, type of discomfort, severity, and factors that cause worsening or lead to improvement. It is important to elucidate whether the symptoms are mainly associated with weight-bearing activities or hip flexion positions.

A complete physical examination should precede the general orthopaedic examination and the dedicated hip examination. Important hip-related tests include evaluation of stance, gait, and limb lengths, as well as a focused neurologic examination that includes lower extremity strength (especially hip abduction), sensation, and coordination. A detailed measurement of passive ranges of hip motion is essential and should include flexion, extension, abduction, adduction, and internal/external rotation in both full extension and 90° of flexion. The anterior impingement test, performed by passively moving the hip into flexion, adduction, and internal rotation, will elicit groin pain in the patient with acetabular rim syndrome secondary to DDH.[19] The anterior apprehension, bicycle, and Patrick (flexion, abduction, and external rotation [FABER]) tests also should be performed.

Imaging

The initial imaging evaluation[47] should include a weight-bearing AP radiograph of the hips and pelvis, with the beam centered on the femoral heads. Acetabular coverage is estimated by measuring the lateral center-edge angle of Wiberg[48] (a normal measurement is >25°) and the acetabular index of Tönnis[49] (a normal measurement is 0° to 10°). Joint subluxation is evaluated by measuring the Shenton line, and acetabular retroversion is evaluated by assessing the crossover sign[50] and the projection of the ischial spine into the pelvis.[51] Although acetabular version is extremely varied in both dysplastic and nondysplastic hips, acetabular retroversion is present in 18% to 30% of adult patients with hip dysplasia.[52,53] A false-profile view (**Figure 2, D**) is also obtained to investigate the anterior coverage of the femoral head by measuring the anterior center-edge angle (a normal measurement is >20°).[54] A Dunn[55] lateral view of the proximal femur provides information about the sphericity of the femoral head and the head-neck offset that may be quantified by measuring the α angle and the head-neck offset ratio.[47] Functional radiographs of the hip in abduction and internal rotation provide additional information by simulating the redirection achieved with a realignment osteotomy. These functional radiographs are needed to confirm the adequacy of gliding femoroacetabular mobility to allow congruous realignment. Acetabular dysplasia, by definition, involves relative undercoverage of the femoral head as assessed using any of the following parameters:[47,49,54] a lateral center-edge angle less than 20°, a Tönnis roof angle (tilt of the sourcil) greater than 20°, coverage less than 80%, an extrusion index greater than 20%, and an anterior center-edge angle less than 20°.

CT and MRI play a role in understanding the biomechanical environment of the hip and estimating the prognosis after surgical intervention.[56] Secondary damage to the labrum and articular cartilage is not demonstrated radiographically and may be severe enough to compromise the results of joint-preserving treatment. CT allows better understanding of the bony anatomy of the pelvis, especially when the pelvis has undergone

prior osteotomies.[57] MRI has been used as a prognostic factor because the delayed gadolinium-enhanced MRI of cartilage (dGEMRIC) technique for examining the dysplastic hip has correlated well with the success of periacetabular osteotomy (PAO).[58] With the dGEMRIC technique, the patient receives an intravenous injection of gadolinium-enhanced contrast material and then is asked to walk for 30 minutes before a multislice fast spin-echo (FSE) sequence is obtained. A dGEMRIC index can be computed that reflects the loss of glycosaminoglycan secondary to degeneration of the articular cartilage.[59]

Interventions for the Adult Patient

In acetabular dysplasia, lack of bone coverage results in instability and superolateral subluxation of the femoral head, which ultimately leads to chronic mechanical overload of the acetabular rim. This overload may ultimately result in degenerative cyst formation, tear or detachment of the acetabular labrum (acetabular rim fracture), and progression of osteoarthritis[19] (**Figure 3**). Isolated treatment of the damaged labrum in a dysplastic hip is not recommended unless the acetabulum is in a stable alignment. In the presence of a dysplastic acetabulum, arthroscopic or open labral débridement or repair must be performed in association with acetabular realignment or the clinical problem will worsen because of the destabilizing effect of the isolated labral procedure.[60] The authors of this chapter prefer to perform an anterior arthrotomy with PAO in patients with a high risk of FAI or labral instability.[61]

Realignment osteotomy of the acetabulum is the principal joint-preserving treatment for acetabular dysplasia, the most common element in developmental dysplasia of the mature hip. Proximal femoral osteotomy alone is usually insufficient for the stabilization of a hip with residual acetabular dysplasia;[62] however, when proximal femoral deformity is present, intertrochanteric osteotomy may be required.[63] A femoral osteotomy may be indicated in conjunction with an acetabular reorientation osteotomy in more severe cases of DDH in the adult.[64,65] Most often, the most appropriate site of correction in the treatment of hip dysplasia in the skeletally mature patient is the periacetabular region.

Various types of pelvic osteotomies have been proposed to reorient the dysplastic acetabulum and nor-

FIGURE 3

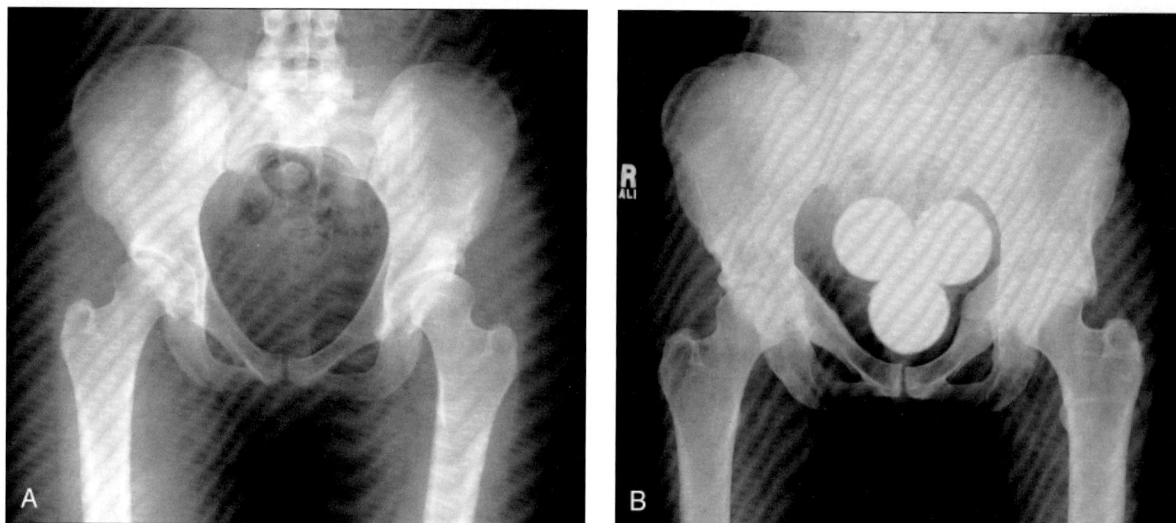

Radiographs of the pelvis of a woman with bilateral hip dysplasia who underwent bilateral periacetabular osteotomy. **A,** Preoperative AP view shows more severe dysplasia in the left hip, characterized by a negative lateral center-edge angle, a break in the Shenton line, and an acetabular rim fracture. **B,** Postoperative AP view obtained at 10-year follow-up shows that the rim fracture in the left hip has healed.

malize the mechanics of the hip. Innominate osteotomy[36] alone is insufficient to restore joint stability in more complex and severe dysplasia in the adult population. Spherical and rotational acetabular osteotomies[66-68] allow excellent coverage of the femoral head. However, the small size of the acetabular fragment makes rigid fixation difficult and hampers early ambulation. In 1988, Ganz et al[69] described the polygon-shaped Bernese PAO, which has the advantage of a relatively large yet mobile acetabular fragment with an excellent blood supply. PAO allows major multiplanar correction and rigid fixation using abductor-sparing approaches, which permit early restoration of function and partial weight bearing with crutches within a few days after surgery.[70] Mechanically, PAO should stabilize the dysplastic hip, which reduces rim loading to physiologic levels and avoids creating FAI. Anatomically, the surgeon should attempt to create a nearly horizontal sourcil and restore the Shenton line on the postoperative AP pelvic radiograph, with no lateralization of the joint center and no retroversion of the acetabulum (no crossover sign or posterior wall sign). In men, because of their generally tight ligaments and more robust osteology, somewhat less correction may better help avoid

postoperative FAI. In the operating room, before closure, impingement-free passive hip flexion to more than 90° should be preserved. If this amount of free flexion is not possible, then either reducing the correction or performing an anterior arthrotomy with anterior femoral head-neck osteochondroplasty should be considered.

PAO has become the most commonly used acetabular reorientation osteotomy in North America and much of Europe for treatment of the mature dysplastic hip.[71-78] Using conversion to total hip arthroplasty as the end point, the hip survival rate at 9 years has been estimated to be 76% to 82%.[74,79] Steppacher et al[76] conducted a study on the mean 20-year follow-up of patients who underwent the Bernese PAO and demonstrated that PAO is an effective technique for treating symptomatic DDH and can maintain the natural hip for at least 19 years in most patients (**Figure 4**). Preoperative risk factors associated with a poor outcome include the presence of advanced arthritis, patient age, a positive impingement test result corresponding to a labral tear, the presence of a limp, and a low Merle d'Aubigné and Postel score.[76] Matheny et al[74] have also identified similar factors, especially age older than 35 years, joint incongruity, and joint space less than 2 mm, as risk fac-

FIGURE 4

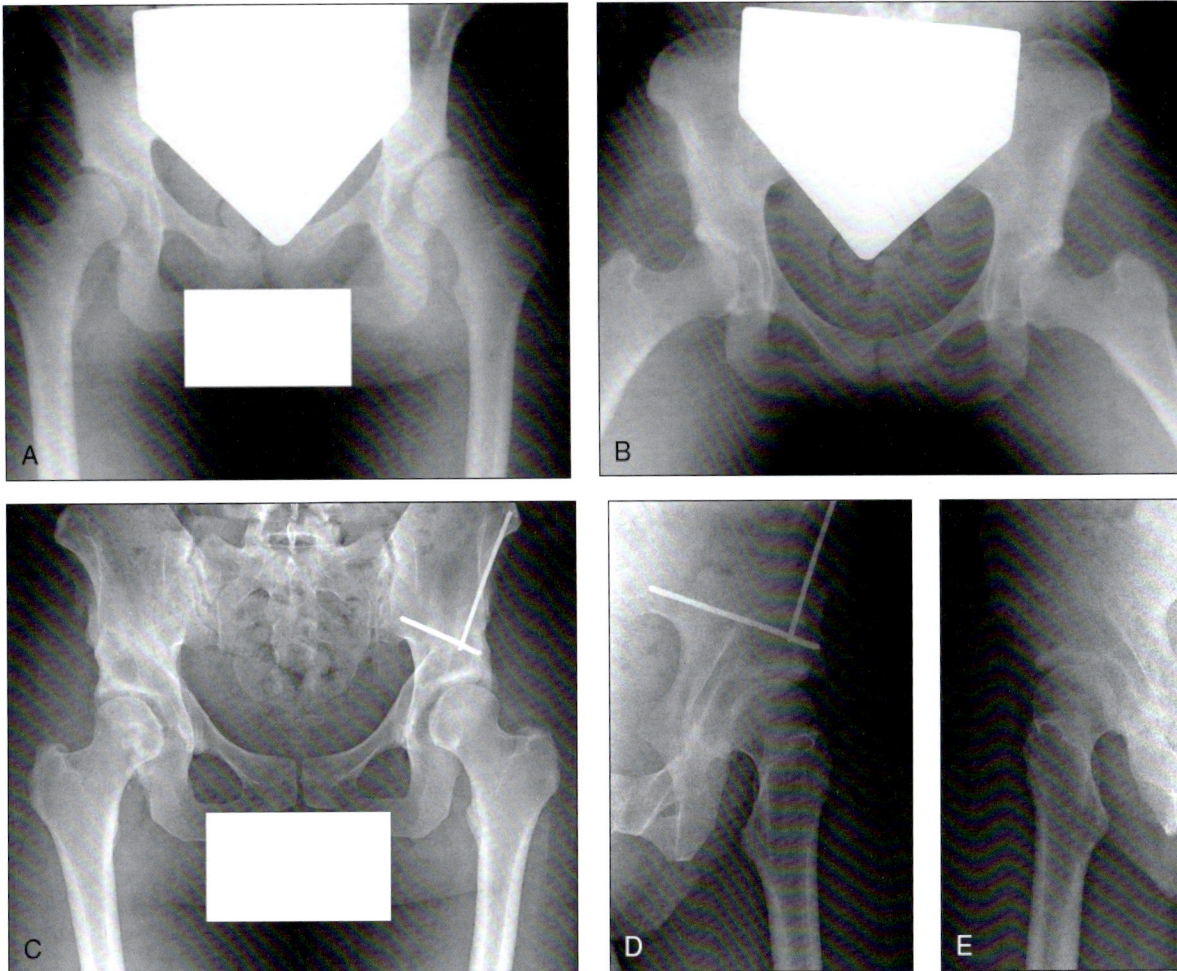

Radiographs of the pelvis of a woman with bilateral hip dysplasia who underwent bilateral periacetabular osteotomy. **A,** Preoperative AP weight-bearing view demonstrates severe acetabular dysplasia, with subluxation of the left hip. **B,** Von Rosen view shows both hips are concentrically reduced. **C,** Postoperative AP weight-bearing view at 7-year follow-up shows that both hips are well reduced, the joints have been medialized, and the sourcil is oriented normally. The joint space is preserved. The Shenton line has been restored in the left hip. Postoperative false-profile views of the left (**D**) and right (**E**) hips demonstrate the restored anterior coverage of the femoral head.

tors for total hip arthroplasty after a PAO.[74] Cunningham et al[58] have also noted that hips that have a higher Tönnis arthritis grade (2 or 3), any joint subluxation, or a lower dGEMRIC index are less likely to benefit from PAO.[58] The rate of complications associated with PAO ranges from 6% to 37% of cases.[72] In general, the risk of complication lessens with the surgeon's experience.

SLIPPED CAPITAL FEMORAL EPIPHYSIS
Incidence
SCFE, the most common hip disorder of adolescent onset, is characterized by an abnormal shearing failure of the capital femoral physis that is usually very gradual, which allows the femoral head to slip posteriorly as the femoral neck and metaphysis move anteriorly and into

external rotation. SCFE affects males more often than females; the mean age at diagnosis is 13.5 years for boys and 12.0 years for girls.[80] Patients with the stable form of SCFE usually present with no history of trauma and a history of gradually increasing knee, thigh, or groin pain, associated with a slight limp and out-toeing gait. Although the stable form is far more common, SCFE also may be unstable, with the patient often acutely unable to bear weight on the involved extremity.[81] At presentation, SCFE is usually unilateral; however, the rate of subsequent contralateral SCFE is high. The overall prevalence of bilateral involvement ranges from 21%[82] to 82%.[83] The incidence varies according to geographic area but has been estimated to be approximately 2 cases per 100,000 persons.[84]

Common Childhood Interventions

SCFE presents two different but related problems to the clinician. First, the open slipping physis must be stabilized or progression of the associated deformity will occur, sometimes acutely, with potentially catastrophic consequences for the blood supply to the femoral head. Second, the deformity associated with even the mildest case of SCFE usually creates a cam-type FAI, which can lead to dysfunction and osteoarthritis even if the physis is stabilized without further slipping.[85]

Treatment of SCFE in childhood and adolescence is determined largely by the stability of the physis and the degree of deformity. SCFE has been classified as acute (<3 weeks of symptoms), chronic (>3 weeks of symptoms), or acute-on-chronic (characterized by exacerbation of pain in a patient who had been symptomatic for more than 3 weeks). Classifying SCFE as stable (patients who are able to walk) or unstable (patients who cannot bear weight, even with crutches) is important, because osteonecrosis of the femoral head has been shown to occur in approximately 50% of patients with unstable SCFE[81] but is extremely rare in patients with stable SCFE.

The primary goal of treatment of SCFE in a patient with an open physis is to stabilize the physis and prevent further slip, while avoiding the complication of osteonecrosis. Indeed, in situ fixation of SCFE has for many years been the standard initial treatment of stable SCFE, no matter how severe the associated deformity, because such stabilization usually leads to closure of the

physis and short-term reliable improvement in function. Consideration of the associated proximal femoral deformity is also clinically important, because cam-type FAI leads to cumulative articular damage in many post-SCFE hips. More emphasis, therefore, has been given to restoration of the normal anatomy of the epiphyseal-metaphyseal junction because residual deformity with a prominent metaphysis has been shown to cause mechanical damage to the acetabular cartilage.[85] The most common treatment options include in situ fixation,[86] closed reduction and percutaneous fixation,[87] fixation associated with primary corrective osteotomy,[88-91] and open reduction with internal fixation.[92-94] Ganz et al[95] described a safe technique for surgical dislocation of the hip that allows full inspection of the joint. The surgical dislocation approach preserves the blood supply to the femoral head and permits complete anatomic reduction under direct visualization.[96,97]

Outcomes

Long-term outcomes following SCFE in adolescence are determined by the success rate following surgical intervention and by the residual deformity at the metaphyseal-epiphyseal junction. Osteonecrosis as a complication of the management of SCFE is known to be associated with osteoarthritis and poor long-term results.[98,99] The risk of late osteoarthritis of the hip is related to the severity of the deformity at skeletal maturity.[100] In a study of patients with untreated SCFE, Carney et al[100] demonstrated that the slip can progress to a severe degree and later result in degenerative arthritis of the hip. For mild untreated SCFE, the long-term results were better than those for more severe SCFE; however, only one third of all patients included had no radiographic evidence of degenerative joint disease. Mild pistol grip[7] or head tilt[5] deformities of the proximal femur were described as sequelae of mild SCFE that may also develop in the contralateral, apparently uninvolved hip and can be associated with late osteoarthritis[7,10] (**Figure 5**). Goodman et al[101] studied human cadaver femora and reported that approximately 70% had severe osteoarthritis in hips with minimum postslip morphology.

Work by Ganz et al has led to a better understanding of the pathophysiology of osteoarthritis in hips with residual deformity secondary to SCFE.[12,102] Proximal femoral deformity secondary to treated or untreated SCFE

FIGURE 5

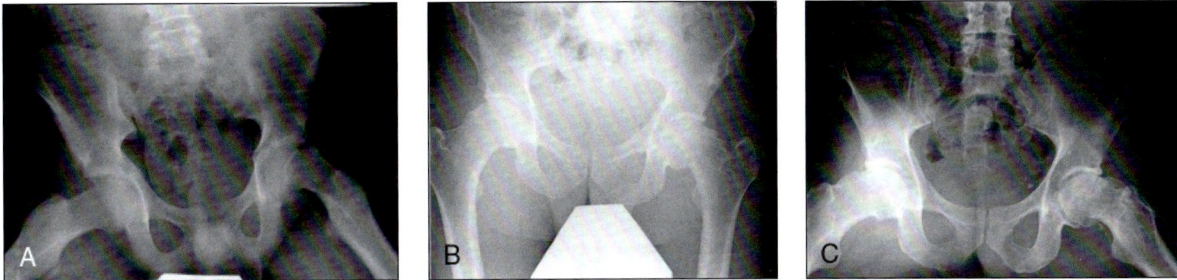

Radiographs of the pelvis of a man with acute slipped capital femoral epiphysis (SCFE) in the left hip who underwent in situ fixation at 11 years of age. **A,** Preoperative frog-lateral view demonstrates SCFE. The right hip was asymptomatic until the patient presented at age 34 years with bilateral hip pain. **B,** AP pelvic view shows the morphology of both hips, with a lack of femoral head-neck offset and the typical pistol grip and hook deformities. **C,** Frog-lateral view shows the deformity at the femoral head-neck junction.

during adolescence is currently accepted as a major cause of cam-type FAI. Reduced anterolateral femoral head-neck offset secondary to SCFE causes the femoral head to impact against the acetabular rim during hip flexion, leading to outside-in chondral abrasion and acetabular labrum detachment, with inevitable secondary osteoarthritis.[2,12,13,102]

Adult Sequelae

Presenting Symptoms

Adult patients with FAI secondary to SCFE typically present with insidious onset of pain in the hip and groin, or sometimes in the buttock, that is exacerbated by activities that require hip flexion, such as sitting.

Evaluation

On physical examination, limited passive hip motion is almost always found, and flexion and internal rotation are particularly limited. Internal rotation is often 0° or less, particularly when tested with the hip in 90° of flexion. The hip classically tends to externally rotate as it is passively flexed. Even if allowed to externally rotate, the involved hip often cannot flex past 90°, and adduction often is less than 0° in this position. The anterior impingement test usually has a positive result: pain is reproduced in the groin when the hip is placed in 90° of flexion and the femur is brought into adduction and internal rotation.[19]

A complete radiographic examination of the hip should include an AP pelvic view, a false-profile view, and a lateral view of the proximal femur. Imaging find-ings can include the mechanically problematic cam deformity of the head-neck junction, in the form of the metaphyseal bump, which is the remodeled anterolateral corner of the proximal femoral neck just distal to the old healed physis. On the AP pelvic radiograph, the depth of the acetabulum can be evaluated using the ilioischial line as a reference: if the floor of the fossa acetabuli touches or is medial to the ilioischial line, the hip is classified as coxa profunda, and if the medial aspect of the femoral head is medial to the ilioischial line, the hip is classified as protrusio acetabuli.[47] Acetabular retroversion can be identified by the presence of the crossover sign[50] and the projection of the ischial spine into the pelvis.[51] On the lateral radiograph of the proximal femur, the angle between the middle axis of the neck and the point where the bone of the head-neck junction crosses outside the radius of curvature of the head (α angle) should be measured. An α angle greater than 50.5° is considered abnormal.[103] CT is useful for better understanding the three dimensions of the deformity and for surgical planning. MRI combined with either gadolinium-based magnetic resonance arthrography or the dGEMRIC[104] technique allows evaluation of the labrum and chondrolabral junction, and should be performed routinely before surgical intervention.

Interventions for the Adult Patient

The surgical treatment of all types of FAI is still somewhat controversial because long-term prospective studies are lacking. As a result, the long-term results of uncorrected, healed SCFE tend to be worse when the deformity is more severe. The long-term results of both intertrochanteric osteotomy[105] and combined cuneiform subcapital wedge resection of the femoral neck and open reduction of the femoral head[93] performed at centers with experienced surgeons seem better than natural history. The Iowa experience,[106,107] in which surgical realignment seemed to lead to worse outcomes than the natural history of the simply stabilized deformity, likely reflects the technically inferior surgical techniques that were available 3 to 5 decades ago, when compared with the contemporary therapeutic armamentarium.

Hip-preserving surgery for the mature hip with a healed SCFE may be indicated for symptoms associated with FAI (**Figure 6**). It is wise to first establish the extent of the damage to the articular surfaces, because the degree of cartilage damage is an important limiting factor in the outcome of hip-preserving techniques for all mechanical disorders of the native hip.

The mechanical principle of joint-preserving treatment of FAI associated with healed SCFE is the elimination of the impingement, either by removing the bump or in some other manner that prevents abnormal contact between the femoral neck and acetabular cartilage. The goals of treatment are to reduce or eliminate symptoms, gain better hip range of motion, and prevent further damage to the chondrolabral junction. The two main categories of surgery for the management of FAI after SCFE are (1) osteochondroplasty of the femoral head-neck junction, sometimes accompanied by acetabular rim trimming if acetabular overcoverage is present; and (2) realignment osteotomy of the proximal femur. Femoral head-neck offset can be restored by using either open or arthroscopic osteochondroplasty[108] of the femoral head-neck junction. Open osteochondroplasty may be performed using an anterior approach[109] and surgical dislocation of the hip joint.[95,110] Realignment osteotomy may be performed in the subcapital,[111,112] basicervical,[88] intertrochanteric,[90] or subtrochanteric region.[91] For severe deformities, correction often requires both osteochondroplasty and osteotomy of the proximal femur.[110,113]

LEGG-CALVÉ-PERTHES DISEASE
Incidence
LCP disease, first described approximately 100 years ago,[114-116] is still considered an idiopathic ischemic necrosis of the growing femoral head. LCP disease has a variable course and can lead to a spectrum of residual deformities of the proximal end of the femur. The incidence of LCP disease varies by geographic region. Ethnic and social factors also are important. The yearly incidence of LCP disease has been reported to range from 1.7 to 15.6 children per 100,000 age 14 years or younger.[117, 118] The estimated incidence of LCP disease in the United States in the 1960s was approximately 6 children per 100,000.[119]

LCP disease is a complex hip problem, and any attempted treatment must consider the different phases, the recognized prognostic factors, and the natural history of the disease. Four radiographic stages of the disease are typically recognized: the initial or necrotic phase, fragmentation, reossification, and the residual phase.[120] Most of the femoral head deformity occurs during the first two phases, and the challenge for the treating orthopaedic surgeon is to decide when and how to intervene. Several classification schemes to quantify the amount of involvement of the femoral head have been proposed.[121-124] The most widely adopted classification includes four categories based on involvement of the lateral third of the femoral head.[122,123,125]

Nonsurgical Treatment
Age at onset of symptoms is considered a major prognostic factor in LCP disease. As a general rule, patients up to 6 years of age tend to have a good prognosis and respond well to nonsurgical intervention.[126,127] Over the years, the containment philosophy has been widely accepted in the management of LCP disease during childhood. Containment is based on the principle that the susceptible femoral head will remodel to the shape of the acetabulum. Nonsurgical management with a cast and/or braces has been used, as well as surgical intervention.

Surgical Treatment
The most common surgical procedures for the treatment of LCP disease in childhood are proximal femoral varus osteotomy and pelvic osteotomies (mainly the Salter osteotomy or a shelf procedure). Although a fair number of retrospective series on LCP disease exist in the literature, strong evidence to support one

FIGURE 6

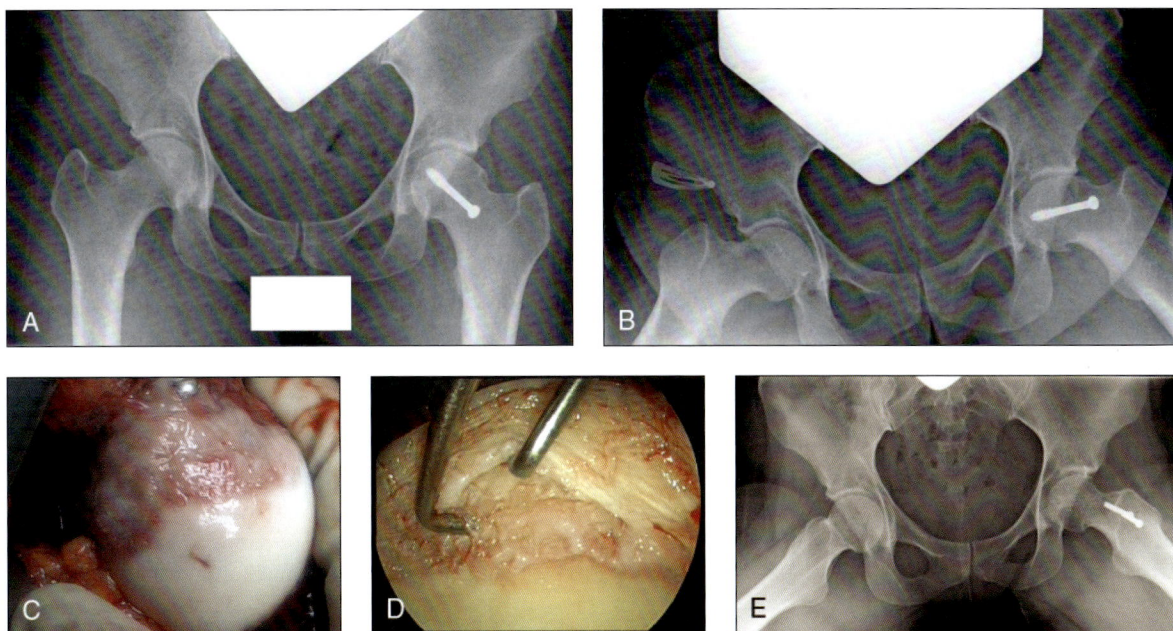

Imaging studies and photographs of the hip of a 27-year-old woman who presented with left hip pain aggravated by activities that require hip flexion. The patient had a history of left slipped capital femoral epiphysis during adolescence that was fixed in situ. AP (**A**) and frog-lateral (**B**) views obtained at presentation show the deformity at the femoral head-neck junction, a cam-type femoroacetabular impingement. **C,** Intraoperative photograph obtained during surgical dislocation of the left hip reveals the severity of the metaphyseal bump. The screw head was also a source of impingement. **D,** Arthroscopic view of the acetabulum reveals delamination of the articular cartilage at the acetabulolabral junction. The labrum was reattached with suture anchors after débridement of the acetabular rim. **E,** Postoperative frog-lateral view demonstrates restored femoral head-neck offset.

specific treatment type is lacking. The strongest level of evidence comes from two multicenter studies. The Perthes Study Group[122,123] showed that children older than 8 years at the time of onset and with a hip in the lateral pillar B group or B/C border group had a better outcome with surgical treatment than with nonsurgical treatment. Children in group B who were younger than 8 years at the time of onset had very favorable outcomes unrelated to treatment, whereas children of all ages in group C frequently had poor outcomes, which also appeared to be unrelated to treatment.[123] A prospective study from Norway reported that children older than 6 years at diagnosis with more than 50% of femoral head involvement had a better outcome after undergoing a proximal femoral varus osteotomy compared with those treated using an orthosis or physical therapy.[127]

Adult Sequelae

LCP disease is associated with a high risk of symptomatic osteoarthritis by middle age. Femoral head deformity and joint congruity are important prognostic factors in the long-term outcome of LCP disease.[128] Stulberg et al[129] classified the radiographic aspects of the hip at skeletal maturity in **Table 1**. Patients with class II hips have a relatively benign long-term prognosis, degenerative joint disease develops in patients with class III and IV hips later in life, and osteoarthritis develops in patients with class V hips early in adulthood.[129,130] In the adolescent or young adult, the hip with prearthritic deformity secondary to LCP disease may not yet be overtly symptomatic. Many patients with a rather severe deformity and limited motion may limit their activities either consciously or unconsciously, which may prevent hip symptoms that otherwise might appear.

TABLE 1 Radiographic Classification of the Hip at Skeletal Maturity

Class	Characteristics
I	Normal hip
II	A spherical femoral head with one of the following: coxa magna, a short femoral neck, or a steep acetabulum
III	A nonspherical but not flat femoral head
IV	A flat femoral head with an abnormal acetabulum (an aspherical congruent hip)
V	A flat femoral head, a normal femoral neck, and a normal acetabulum (an aspherical incongruent hip)

Data adapted from Stulberg SD, Cooperman DR, Wallensten R: The natural history of Legg-Calvé-Perthes disease. *J Bone Joint Surg Am* 1981;63(7):1095-1108.

Presenting Symptoms

Hip deformity after LCP disease has many forms and causes a variety of problematic mechanical abnormalities. Usually, patients with growth disturbances of the proximal femur, including a nonspherical femoral head with a short femoral neck and an overriding greater trochanter, present with symptoms caused by changes in the mechanics of the hip. Deformities secondary to LCP disease are unique in that the hip can demonstrate features of instability in upright activities (for example, walking and running) and yet still cause impingement in hip flexion because of an aspherical femoral head. FAI in LCP disease can be caused by the aspherical femoral head (cam-type FAI) but also may be secondary to acetabular overcoverage due to a retroverted acetabulum[131,132] (pincer-type FAI) and functional retroversion of the articulating portion of the femoral head.[133] In addition, FAI may be extra-articular, secondary to greater trochanter overgrowth or, rarely, because of the proximal position of the lesser trochanter caused by a short femoral neck. Therefore, clinical presentation is similar to that of patients with FAI, who cannot tolerate activities that require hip flexion (for example, sitting). However, if the acetabulum is shallow, then clinical symptoms related to instability, such as groin pain after upright activities, may be present.

Evaluation

Radiographic evaluation is similar to that in patients with FAI secondary to SCFE. Advanced preoperative imaging, including CT and MRI, are important to determine the most spherical portion of the femoral head, which is usually posteromedial, to plan the reconstruction. MRI (dGEMRIC or magnetic resonance arthrography) is advantageous because it allows evaluation of the acetabular labrum.

Interventions for the Adult Patient

The ultimate goal of the treatment of young adults with FAI secondary to LCP disease is to improve impingement-free range of motion and restore joint congruency and stability. Preoperative planning should focus on recognizing the deformities that contribute to the patient's symptoms to differentiate patients with isolated FAI from patients with secondary acetabular dysplasia and instability, and the association of both. Recognizing the source of the impingement (acetabular versus femoral; intra-articular versus extra-articular) between the femoral head-neck junction and the acetabular rim is also required for surgical planning.

The most widely used surgical interventions for the proximal femur include intertrochanteric osteotomy,[63,134] relative femoral neck lengthening,[135] true femoral neck lengthening,[136] and osteochondroplasty of the femoral head-neck junction.[12] Femoral head reduction osteotomy was described recently for correction of an enlarged femoral head;[137] however, long-term results of this procedure are pending. On the acetabular side, extra-articular procedures include redirectional PAOs and acetabular augmentation procedures (for example,

FIGURE 7

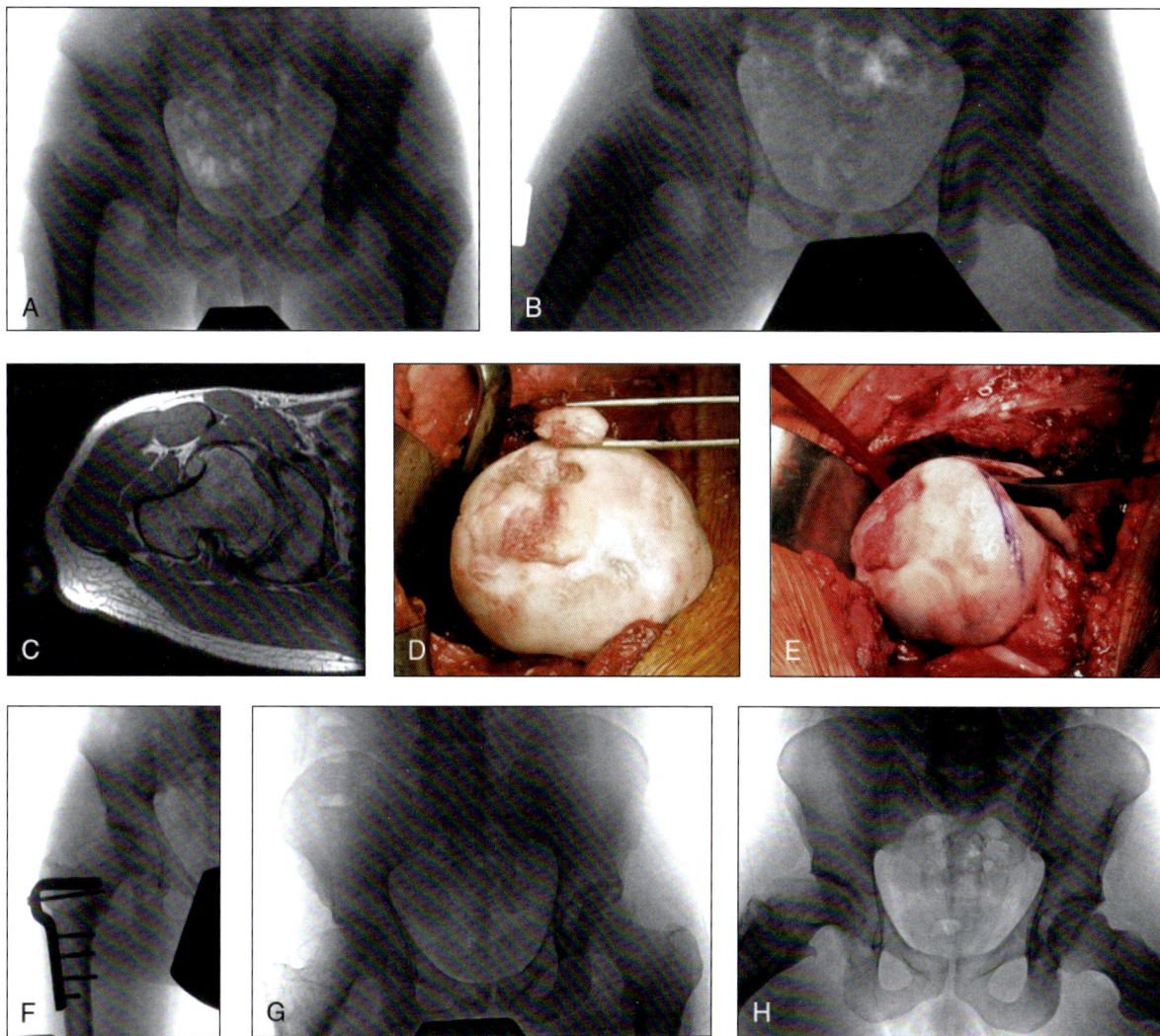

Imaging studies and photographs of the femoral head in a 15-year-old boy with healed Legg-Calvé-Perthes disease who presented with pain after the football season. AP (**A**) and frog-lateral (**B**) radiographs reveal a severe deformity: an aspherical femoral head with a high-rising greater trochanter and a short, thick femoral neck. **C,** Axial oblique MRI reveals a severely misshapen femoral head, a large portion of which is extra-articular. Intraoperative photographs obtained at the time of surgical dislocation of the hip show a loose fragment from the articular portion of the femoral head (**D**) and resection of the portion of the head responsible for extra-articular impingement (**E**). **F,** Postoperative AP view following surgical dislocation of the hip, osteochondroplasty of the femoral head-neck junction, relative lengthening of the greater trochanter and a flexion-valgus proximal femoral osteotomy. Weight-bearing AP (**G**) and frog-lateral (**H**) views obtained at 6-year follow-up show improved femoral head-neck offset and joint congruency.

the shelf procedure), whereas intra-articular procedures include acetabular trimming with labral refixation.[138,139] Complex deformities of the femoral head combined with acetabular dysplasia may require a combined approach.[140] The surgical dislocation approach[95] allows dynamic assessment of the relationship of the femoral head to the acetabulum. Surgical treatment should start with correction of the femoral deformity using this approach (**Figure 7**).

CONCLUSION

Even with optimal treatment before skeletal maturity, developmental hip conditions may result in imperfect hip mechanics at skeletal maturity. Although a prearthritic hip deformity secondary to DDH, healed LCP disease, or healed SCFE may be only mildly symptomatic into early adulthood, most hips with osteoarthritis treated using arthroplasty have one of the developmental deformities discussed earlier in the chapter as the primary etiology. Instability and FAI are now accepted as the major mechanical factors contributing to osteoarthritis. This type of secondary osteoarthritis often becomes symptomatic at too young an age for arthroplasty to be a satisfying choice. Therefore, optimizing the results of primary treatment of pediatric hip conditions is worthwhile, as is the diagnosis and aggressive hip-preserving treatment of any residual deformity in the young adult.

REFERENCES

1. Bombelli R, Santore RF, Poss R: Mechanics of the normal and osteoarthritic hip: A new perspective. *Clin Orthop Relat Res* 1984(182):69-78.

2. Ganz R, Leunig M, Leunig-Ganz K, Harris WH: The etiology of osteoarthritis of the hip: An integrated mechanical concept. *Clin Orthop Relat Res* 2008;466(2):264-272.

3. Aronson J: Osteoarthritis of the young adult hip: Etiology and treatment. *Instr Course Lect* 1986;35:119-128.

4. Cooperman DR, Emery H, Keller C: Factors relating to hip joint arthritis following three childhood diseases—juvenile rheumatoid arthritis, Perthes disease, and postreduction avascular necrosis in congenital hip dislocation. *J Pediatr Orthop* 1986;6(6):706-712.

5. Murray RO: The aetiology of primary osteoarthritis of the hip. *Br J Radiol* 1965;38(455):810-824.

6. Solomon L, Schnitzler CM, Browett JP: Osteoarthritis of the hip: The patient behind the disease. *Ann Rheum Dis* 1982;41(2):118-125.

7. Stulberg SD, Cordell LD, Harris WH, Ramsey PL, MacEwen GD: Unrecognized childhood hip disease: A major cause of idiopathic osteoarthritis of the hip. Paper presented at the Third Open Scientific Meeting of the Hip Society. St. Louis, MO, 1975.

8. Lloyd-Roberts GC: Osteoarthritis of the hip; a study of the clinical pathology. *J Bone Joint Surg Br* 1955; 37-B(1):8-47.

9. Stulberg SD, Harris WH: Acetabular dysplasia and the development of osteoarthritis of the hip. Paper presented at the Second Open Scientific Meeting of the Hip Society. St. Louis, MO, 1974.

10. Solomon L: Patterns of osteoarthritis of the hip. *J Bone Joint Surg Br* 1976;58(2):176-183.

11. Harris WH: Etiology of osteoarthritis of the hip. *Clin Orthop Relat Res* 1986(213):20-33.

12. Ganz R, Parvizi J, Beck M, Leunig M, Nötzli H, Siebenrock KA: Femoroacetabular impingement: A cause for osteoarthritis of the hip. *Clin Orthop Relat Res* 2003(417):112-120.

13. Beck M, Kalhor M, Leunig M, Ganz R: Hip morphology influences the pattern of damage to the acetabular cartilage: Femoroacetabular impingement as a cause of early osteoarthritis of the hip. *J Bone Joint Surg Br* 2005;87(7):1012-1018.

14. Leunig M, Beck M, Dora C, Ganz R: Femoroazetabuläres Impingement als Auslöser der Koxarthrose. *Orthopade* 2006;35(1):77-84.

15. Hack K, Di Primio G, Rakhra K, Beaulé PE: Prevalence of cam-type femoroacetabular impingement morphology in asymptomatic volunteers. *J Bone Joint Surg Am* 2010;92(14):2436-2444.

16. Reichenbach S, Jüni P, Werlen S, et al: Prevalence of cam-type deformity on hip magnetic resonance imaging in young males: A cross-sectional study. *Arthritis Care Res (Hoboken)* 2010;62(9):1319-1327.

17. Pauwels F: *Biomechanics of the Normal and Diseased Hip: Theoretical Foundation, Technique and Results of Treatment. An Atlas.* New York, NY, Springer, 1976.

18. Bombelli R: *Structure and Function in Normal and Abnormal Hips: How to Rescue Mechanically Jeopardized Hips,* ed 3. New York, NY, Springer-Verlag, 1993.

19. Klaue K, Durnin CW, Ganz R: The acetabular rim syndrome: A clinical presentation of dysplasia of the hip. *J Bone Joint Surg Br* 1991;73(3):423-429.

20. Millis MB, Kim YJ: Rationale of osteotomy and related procedures for hip preservation: A review. *Clin Orthop Relat Res* 2002(405):108-121.

21. Coleman SS: Congenital dysplasia of the hip in the Navajo infant. *Clin Orthop Relat Res* 1968(56): 179-193.

22. American Academy of Pediatrics: Clinical practice guideline: Early detection of developmental dysplasia of the hip. Committee on Quality Improvement, Subcommittee on Developmental Dysplasia of the Hip. *Pediatrics* 2000;105(4 Pt 1):896-905.

23. Bialik V, Bialik GM, Blazer S, Sujov P, Wiener F, Berant M: Developmental dysplasia of the hip: A new approach to incidence. *Pediatrics* 1999;103(1):93-99.

24. Noritake K, Yoshihashi Y, Hattori T, Miura T: Acetabular development after closed reduction of congenital dislocation of the hip. *J Bone Joint Surg Br* 1993;75(5):737-743.

25. Schoenecker PL, Dollard PA, Sheridan JJ, Strecker WB: Closed reduction of developmental dislocation of the hip in children older than 18 months. *J Pediatr Orthop* 1995;15(6):763-767.

26. Zionts LE, MacEwen GD: Treatment of congenital dislocation of the hip in children between the ages of one and three years. *J Bone Joint Surg Am* 1986;68(6):829-846.

27. Mardam-Bey TH, MacEwen GD: Congenital hip dislocation after walking age. *J Pediatr Orthop* 1982;2(5):478-486.

28. Ferguson AB Jr: Primary open reduction of congenital dislocation of the hip using a median adductor approach. *J Bone Joint Surg Am* 1973;55(4):671-689.

29. Ludloff L: The open reduction of the congenital hip dislocation by an anterior incision. *Am J Orthop Surg* 1913;10:438-454.

30. Mau H, Dörr WM, Henkel L, Lutsche J: Open reduction of congenital dislocation of the hip by Ludloff's method. *J Bone Joint Surg Am* 1971;53(7):1281-1288.

31. Weinstein SL, Ponseti IV: Congenital dislocation of the hip. *J Bone Joint Surg Am* 1979;61(1):119-124.

32. Morcuende JA, Meyer MD, Dolan LA, Weinstein SL: Long-term outcome after open reduction through an anteromedial approach for congenital dislocation of the hip. *J Bone Joint Surg Am* 1997;79(6):810-817.

33. Klisic P, Jankovic L: Combined procedure of open reduction and shortening of the femur in treatment of congenital dislocation of the hips in older children. *Clin Orthop Relat Res* 1976(119):60-69.

34. Albinana J, Dolan LA, Spratt KF, Morcuende J, Meyer MD, Weinstein SL: Acetabular dysplasia after treatment for developmental dysplasia of the hip: Implications for secondary procedures. *J Bone Joint Surg Br* 2004;86(6):876-886.

35. Kasser JR, Bowen JR, MacEwen GD: Varus derotation osteotomy in the treatment of persistent dysplasia in congenital dislocation of the hip. *J Bone Joint Surg Am* 1985;67(2):195-202.

36. Salter RB: Role of innominate osteotomy in the treatment of congenital dislocation and subluxation of the hip in the older child. *J Bone Joint Surg Am* 1966;48(7):1413-1439.

37. Pemberton PA: Pericapsular osteotomy of the ilium for treatment of congenital subluxation and dislocation of the hip. *J Bone Joint Surg Am* 1965;47:65-86.

38. Weinstein SL, Mubarak SJ, Wenger DR: Developmental hip dysplasia and dislocation: Part II. *Instr Course Lect* 2004;53:531-542.

39. Thomas SR, Wedge JH, Salter RB: Outcome at forty-five years after open reduction and innominate osteotomy for late-presenting developmental dislocation of the hip. *J Bone Joint Surg Am* 2007;89(11):2341-2350.

40. Wedge JH, Thomas SR, Salter RB: Outcome at forty-five years after open reduction and innominate osteotomy for late-presenting developmental dislocation of the hip: Surgical technique. *J Bone Joint Surg Am* 2008;90(Suppl 2 Pt 2):238-253.

41. Weinstein SL: Natural history of congenital hip dislocation (CDH) and hip dysplasia. *Clin Orthop Relat Res* 1987(225):62-76.

42. Dega W: Osteotomia trans-iliakalna w leczeniu wrodzonej dysplazji biodra. *Chir Narzadow Ruchu Ortop Pol* 1974;39(5):601-613.

43. Grudziak JS, Ward WT: Dega osteotomy for the treatment of congenital dysplasia of the hip. *J Bone Joint Surg Am* 2001;83-A(6):845-854.

44. Dora C, Mascard E, Mladenov K, Seringe R: Retroversion of the acetabular dome after Salter and triple pelvic osteotomy for congenital dislocation of the hip. *J Pediatr Orthop B* 2002;11(1):34-40.

45. Murphy SB, Ganz R, Müller ME: The prognosis in untreated dysplasia of the hip: A study of radiographic factors that predict the outcome. *J Bone Joint Surg Am* 1995;77(7):985-989.

46. Cooperman DR, Wallensten R, Stulberg SD: Acetabular dysplasia in the adult. *Clin Orthop Relat Res* 1983(175):79-85.

47. Clohisy JC, Carlisle JC, Beaulé PE, et al: A systematic approach to the plain radiographic evaluation of the

young adult hip. *J Bone Joint Surg Am* 2008;90 (Suppl 4):47-66.

48. Wiberg G: Studies on dysplastic acetabula and congenital subluxation of the hip joint: With special reference to the complication of osteoarthritis. *Acta Chir Scand* 1939;83(Suppl 58):28-38.

49. Tönnis D: *Congenital Dysplasia and Dislocation of the Hip in Children and Adults*. New York, NY, Springer, 1987.

50. Jamali AA, Mladenov K, Meyer DC, et al: Anteroposterior pelvic radiographs to assess acetabular retroversion: High validity of the "cross-over-sign". *J Orthop Res* 2007;25(6):758-765.

51. Kalberer F, Sierra RJ, Madan SS, Ganz R, Leunig M: Ischial spine projection into the pelvis: A new sign for acetabular retroversion. *Clin Orthop Relat Res* 2008;466(3):677-683.

52. Troelsen A, Rømer L, Jacobsen S, Ladelund S, Søballe K: Cranial acetabular retroversion is common in developmental dysplasia of the hip as assessed by the weight bearing position. *Acta Orthop* 2010;81(4):436-441.

53. Fujii M, Nakashima Y, Yamamoto T, et al: Acetabular retroversion in developmental dysplasia of the hip. *J Bone Joint Surg Am* 2010;92(4):895-903.

54. Lequesne M; de SEZE: False profile of the pelvis: A new radiographic incidence for the study of the hip. Its use in dysplasias and different coxopathies. *Rev Rhum Mal Osteoartic* 1961;28:643-652.

55. Dunn DM: Anteversion of the neck of the femur; a method of measurement. *J Bone Joint Surg Br* 1952; 34-B(2):181-186.

56. Leunig M, Podeszwa D, Beck M, Werlen S, Ganz R: Magnetic resonance arthrography of labral disorders in hips with dysplasia and impingement. *Clin Orthop Relat Res* 2004(418):74-80.

57. Millis MB, Murphy SB: Use of computed tomographic reconstruction in planning osteotomies of the hip. *Clin Orthop Relat Res* 1992(274):154-159.

58. Cunningham T, Jessel R, Zurakowski D, Millis MB, Kim YJ: Delayed gadolinium-enhanced magnetic resonance imaging of cartilage to predict early failure of Bernese periacetabular osteotomy for hip dysplasia. *J Bone Joint Surg Am* 2006;88(7):1540-1548.

59. Kim YJ, Jaramillo D, Millis MB, Gray ML, Burstein D: Assessment of early osteoarthritis in hip dysplasia with delayed gadolinium-enhanced magnetic resonance imaging of cartilage. *J Bone Joint Surg Am* 2003; 85-A(10):1987-1992.

60. Wenger DE, Kendell KR, Miner MR, Trousdale RT: Acetabular labral tears rarely occur in the absence of bony abnormalities. *Clin Orthop Relat Res* 2004(426):145-150.

61. Millis MB, Murphy SB: Das Bostoner Konzept: Die periazetabuläre Osteotomie mit simultaner Arthrotomie über den direkten vorderen Zugang. *Orthopade* 1998;27(11):751-758.

62. Perlau R, Wilson MG, Poss R: Isolated proximal femoral osteotomy for treatment of residua of congenital dysplasia or idiopathic osteoarthrosis of the hip: Five to ten-year results. *J Bone Joint Surg Am* 1996;78(10): 1462-1467.

63. Schatzker J: *The Intertrochanteric Osteotomy*. New York, NY, Springer, 1984.

64. Clohisy JC, St John LC, Nunley RM, Schutz AL, Schoenecker PL: Combined periacetabular and femoral osteotomies for severe hip deformities. *Clin Orthop Relat Res* 2009;467(9):2221-2227.

65. Clohisy JC, Barrett SE, Gordon JE, Delgado ED, Schoenecker PL: Periacetabular osteotomy in the treatment of severe acetabular dysplasia: Surgical technique. *J Bone Joint Surg Am* 2006;88(Suppl 1 Pt 1):65-83.

66. Nishio A: Transposition osteotomy of the acetabulum in the treatment of congenital dislocation of the hip. *J Jpn Ortho Assoc* 1956;30:483.

67. Ninomiya S, Tagawa H: Rotational acetabular osteotomy for the dysplastic hip. *J Bone Joint Surg Am* 1984;66(3):430-436.

68. Wagner H: Osteotomies for congenital hip dislocation. Paper presented at the Fourth Open Scientific Meeting of the Hip Society. St. Louis, MO, 1976.

69. Ganz R, Klaue K, Vinh TS, Mast JW: A new periacetabular osteotomy for the treatment of hip dysplasias: Technique and preliminary results. *Clin Orthop Relat Res* 1988(232):26-36.

70. Murphy SB, Millis MB: Periacetabular osteotomy without abductor dissection using direct anterior exposure. *Clin Orthop Relat Res* 1999(364):92-98.

71. Clohisy JC, Barrett SE, Gordon JE, Delgado ED, Schoenecker PL: Periacetabular osteotomy for the treatment of severe acetabular dysplasia. *J Bone Joint Surg Am* 2005;87(2):254-259.

72. Clohisy JC, Schutz AL, St John L, Schoenecker PL, Wright RW: Periacetabular osteotomy: A systematic

literature review. *Clin Orthop Relat Res* 2009;467(8): 2041-2052.

73. Leunig M, Siebenrock KA, Ganz R: Rationale of periacetabular osteotomy and background work. *Instr Course Lect* 2001;50:229-238.

74. Matheney T, Kim YJ, Zurakowski D, Matero C, Millis M: Intermediate to long-term results following the Bernese periacetabular osteotomy and predictors of clinical outcome. *J Bone Joint Surg Am* 2009;91(9):2113-2123.

75. Millis MB, Kain M, Sierra R, et al: Periacetabular osteotomy for acetabular dysplasia in patients older than 40 years: A preliminary study. *Clin Orthop Relat Res* 2009;467(9):2228-2234.

76. Steppacher SD, Tannast M, Ganz R, Siebenrock KA: Mean 20-year followup of Bernese periacetabular osteotomy. *Clin Orthop Relat Res* 2008;466(7):1633-1644.

77. Trousdale RT, Ekkernkamp A, Ganz R, Wallrichs SL: Periacetabular and intertrochanteric osteotomy for the treatment of osteoarthrosis in dysplastic hips. *J Bone Joint Surg Am* 1995;77(1):73-85.

78. Siebenrock KA, Schöll E, Lottenbach M, Ganz R: Bernese periacetabular osteotomy. *Clin Orthop Relat Res* 1999(363):9-20.

79. Troelsen A, Elmengaard B, Søballe K: Medium-term outcome of periacetabular osteotomy and predictors of conversion to total hip replacement. *J Bone Joint Surg Am* 2009;91(9):2169-2179.

80. Loder RT: The demographics of slipped capital femoral epiphysis: An international multicenter study. *Clin Orthop Relat Res* 1996(322):8-27.

81. Loder RT, Richards BS, Shapiro PS, Reznick LR, Aronson DD: Acute slipped capital femoral epiphysis: The importance of physeal stability. *J Bone Joint Surg Am* 1993;75(8):1134-1140.

82. Hägglund G, Hansson LI, Ordeberg G: Epidemiology of slipped capital femoral epiphysis in southern Sweden. *Clin Orthop Relat Res* 1984(191):82-94.

83. Loder RT, Aronson DD, Greenfield ML: The epidemiology of bilateral slipped capital femoral epiphysis: A study of children in Michigan. *J Bone Joint Surg Am* 1993;75(8):1141-1147.

84. Crawford AH: Slipped capital femoral epiphysis. *J Bone Joint Surg Am* 1988;70(9):1422-1427.

85. Leunig M, Casillas MM, Hamlet M, et al: Slipped capital femoral epiphysis: Early mechanical damage to the acetabular cartilage by a prominent femoral metaphysis. *Acta Orthop Scand* 2000;71(4):370-375.

86. Aronson DD, Peterson DA, Miller DV: Slipped capital femoral epiphysis: The case for internal fixation in situ. *Clin Orthop Relat Res* 1992(281):115-122.

87. Fahey JJ, O'Brien ET: acute slipped capital femoral epiphysis: Review of the literature and report of ten cases. *J Bone Joint Surg Am* 1965;47:1105-1127.

88. Barmada R, Bruch RF, Gimbel JS, Ray RD: Base of the neck extracapsular osteotomy for correction of deformity in slipped capital femoral epiphysis. *Clin Orthop Relat Res* 1978(132):98-101.

89. Dunn DM: The treatment of adolescent slipping of the upper femoral epiphysis. *J Bone Joint Surg Br* 1964;46:621-629.

90. Imhäuser G: Zur Pathogenese und Therapie der jugendlichen Hüftkopflösung. *Z Orthop Ihre Grenzgeb* 1957;88:3-41.

91. Southwick WO: Osteotomy through the lesser trochanter for slipped capital femoral epiphysis. *J Bone Joint Surg Am* 1967;49(5):807-835.

92. Parsch K, Weller S, Parsch D: Open reduction and smooth Kirschner wire fixation for unstable slipped capital femoral epiphysis. *J Pediatr Orthop* 2009;29(1): 1-8.

93. Velasco R, Schai PA, Exner GU: Slipped capital femoral epiphysis: A long-term follow-up study after open reduction of the femoral head combined with subcapital wedge resection. *J Pediatr Orthop B* 1998;7(1): 43-52.

94. Broughton NS, Todd RC, Dunn DM, Angel JC: Open reduction of the severely slipped upper femoral epiphysis. *J Bone Joint Surg Br* 1988;70(3):435-439.

95. Ganz R, Gill TJ, Gautier E, Ganz K, Krügel N, Berlemann U: Surgical dislocation of the adult hip a technique with full access to the femoral head and acetabulum without the risk of avascular necrosis. *J Bone Joint Surg Br* 2001;83(8):1119-1124.

96. Leunig M, Slongo T, Kleinschmidt M, Ganz R: Subcapital correction osteotomy in slipped capital femoral epiphysis by means of surgical hip dislocation. *Oper Orthop Traumatol* 2007;19(4):389-410.

97. Ziebarth K, Zilkens C, Spencer S, Leunig M, Ganz R, Kim YJ: Capital realignment for moderate and severe SCFE using a modified Dunn procedure. *Clin Orthop Relat Res* 2009;467(3):704-716.

98. Rattey T, Piehl F, Wright JG: Acute slipped capital femoral epiphysis: Review of outcomes and rates of avascular necrosis. *J Bone Joint Surg Am* 1996;78(3):398-402.

99. Krahn TH, Canale ST, Beaty JH, Warner WC, Lourenço P: Long-term follow-up of patients with avascular necrosis after treatment of slipped capital femoral epiphysis. *J Pediatr Orthop* 1993;13(2):154-158.

100. Carney BT, Weinstein SL, Noble J: Long-term follow-up of slipped capital femoral epiphysis. *J Bone Joint Surg Am* 1991;73(5):667-674.

101. Goodman DA, Feighan JE, Smith AD, Latimer B, Buly RL, Cooperman DR: Subclinical slipped capital femoral epiphysis: Relationship to osteoarthrosis of the hip. *J Bone Joint Surg Am* 1997;79(10):1489-1497.

102. Leunig M, Beaulé PE, Ganz R: The concept of femoroacetabular impingement: Current status and future perspectives. *Clin Orthop Relat Res* 2009;467(3):616-622.

103. Beaulé PE, Allen DJ, Clohisy JC, Schoenecker PL, Leunig M: The young adult with hip impingement: Deciding on the optimal intervention. *Instr Course Lect* 2009;58:213-222.

104. Zilkens C, Miese F, Bittersohl B, et al: Delayed gadolinium-enhanced magnetic resonance imaging of cartilage (dGEMRIC), after slipped capital femoral epiphysis. *Eur J Radiol* 2011;79(3):400-406.

105. Schai PA, Exner GU, Hänsch O: Prevention of secondary coxarthrosis in slipped capital femoral epiphysis: A long-term follow-up study after corrective intertrochanteric osteotomy. *J Pediatr Orthop B* 1996;5(3):135-143.

106. Dobbs MB, Weinstein SL: Natural history and long-term outcomes of slipped capital femoral epiphysis. *Instr Course Lect* 2001;50:571-575.

107. Carney BT, Weinstein SL: Natural history of untreated chronic slipped capital femoral epiphysis. *Clin Orthop Relat Res* 1996(322):43-47.

108. Ilizaliturri VM Jr, Nossa-Barrera JM, Acosta-Rodriguez E, Camacho-Galindo J: Arthroscopic treatment of femoroacetabular impingement secondary to paediatric hip disorders. *J Bone Joint Surg Br* 2007;89(8):1025-1030.

109. Herndon CH, Heyman CH, Bell DM: Treatment of slipped capital femoral epiphysis by epiphyseodesis and osteoplasty of the femoral neck: A report of further experiences. *J Bone Joint Surg Am* 1963;45:999-1012.

110. Spencer S, Millis MB, Kim YJ: Early results of treatment of hip impingement syndrome in slipped capital femoral epiphysis and pistol grip deformity of the femoral head-neck junction using the surgical dislocation technique. *J Pediatr Orthop* 2006;26(3):281-285.

111. Dunn DM, Angel JC: Replacement of the femoral head by open operation in severe adolescent slipping of the upper femoral epiphysis. *J Bone Joint Surg Br* 1978;60-B(3):394-403.

112. Fish JB: Cuneiform osteotomy of the femoral neck in the treatment of slipped capital femoral epiphysis. *J Bone Joint Surg Am* 1984;66(8):1153-1168.

113. Rebello G, Spencer S, Millis MB, Kim YJ: Surgical dislocation in the management of pediatric and adolescent hip deformity. *Clin Orthop Relat Res* 2009;467(3):724-731.

114. Calvé J: Sur une forme particulière de pseudo-coxalgie greffée sur des déformations caractéristiques de l'extrémité supérieure du fémur. *Rev Chir* 1910;42:54-84.

115. Legg AT: An obscure affection of the hip-joint. *Boston Med Surg J* 1910;162:202-204.

116. Perthes G: Über arthritis deformans juvenilis. *Deutsche Zeitschr Chir* 1910(107):111-159.

117. Purry NA: The incidence of Perthes' disease in three population groups in the Eastern Cape region of South Africa. *J Bone Joint Surg Br* 1982;64(3):286-288.

118. Barker DJ, Hall AJ: The epidemiology of Perthes' disease. *Clin Orthop Relat Res* 1986(209):89-94.

119. Molloy MK, MacMahon B: Incidence of Legg-Perthes disease (osteochondritis deformans). *N Engl J Med* 1966;275(18):988-990.

120. Waldenström H: The definitive forms of coxa plana. *Acta Radiol* 1922;1:384.

121. Catterall A: Legg-Calvé-Perthes syndrome. *Clin Orthop Relat Res* 1981(158):41-52.

122. Herring JA, Kim HT, Browne R: Legg-Calve-Perthes disease: Part I. Classification of radiographs with use of the modified lateral pillar and Stulberg classifications. *J Bone Joint Surg Am* 2004;86-A(10):2103-2120.

123. Herring JA, Kim HT, Browne R: Legg-Calve-Perthes disease: Part II. Prospective multicenter study of the effect of treatment on outcome. *J Bone Joint Surg Am* 2004;86-A(10):2121-2134.

124. Salter RB, Thompson GH: Legg-Calvé-Perthes disease: The prognostic significance of the subchondral fracture and a two-group classification of the femoral head involvement. *J Bone Joint Surg Am* 1984;66(4):479-489.

125. Herring JA, Neustadt JB, Williams JJ, Early JS, Browne RH: The lateral pillar classification of Legg-Calvé-Perthes disease. *J Pediatr Orthop* 1992;12(2):143-150.

126. Rosenfeld SB, Herring JA, Chao JC: Legg-calve-perthes disease: A review of cases with onset before six years of age. *J Bone Joint Surg Am* 2007;89(12):2712-2722.

127. Wiig O, Terjesen T, Svenningsen S: Prognostic factors and outcome of treatment in Perthes' disease: A prospective study of 368 patients with five-year follow-up. *J Bone Joint Surg Br* 2008;90(10):1364-1371.

128. Sponseller PD, Desai SS, Millis MB: Abnormalities of proximal femoral growth after severe Perthes' disease. *J Bone Joint Surg Br* 1989;71(4):610-614.

129. Stulberg SD, Cooperman DR, Wallensten R: The natural history of Legg-Calvé-Perthes disease. *J Bone Joint Surg Am* 1981;63(7):1095-1108.

130. Ippolito E, Tudisco C, Farsetti P: The long-term prognosis of unilateral Perthes' disease. *J Bone Joint Surg Br* 1987;69(2):243-250.

131. Sankar WN, Flynn JM: The development of acetabular retroversion in children with Legg-Calvé-Perthes disease. *J Pediatr Orthop* 2008;28(4):440-443.

132. Eijer H: Towards a better understanding of the aetiology of Legg-Calvé-Perthes' disease: Acetabular retroversion may cause abnormal loading of dorsal femoral head-neck junction with restricted blood supply to the femoral epiphysis. *Med Hypotheses* 2007;68(5):995-997.

133. Kim HT, Wenger DR: "Functional retroversion" of the femoral head in Legg-Calvé-Perthes disease and epiphyseal dysplasia: Analysis of head-neck deformity and its effect on limb position using three-dimensional computed tomography. *J Pediatr Orthop* 1997;17(2):240-246.

134. Millis MB, Murphy SB, Poss R: Osteotomies about the hip for the prevention and treatment of osteoarthrosis. *Instr Course Lect* 1996;45:209-226.

135. Ganz R, Huff TW, Leunig M: Extended retinacular soft-tissue flap for intra-articular hip surgery: Surgical technique, indications, and results of application. *Instr Course Lect* 2009;58:241-255.

136. Lascombes P, Prevot J, Allouche A, Ligier JN, Metaizeau JP: Lengthening osteotomy of the femoral neck with transposition of the greater trochanter in acquired coxa vara. *Rev Chir Orthop Reparatrice Appar Mot* 1985;71(8):599-601.

137. Ganz R, Horowitz K, Leunig M: Algorithm for femoral and periacetabular osteotomies in complex hip deformities. *Clin Orthop Relat Res* 2010;468(12):3168-3180.

138. Espinosa N, Beck M, Rothenfluh DA, Ganz R, Leunig M: Treatment of femoro-acetabular impingement: preliminary results of labral refixation: Surgical technique. *J Bone Joint Surg Am* 2007;89(Suppl 2 Pt 1):36-53.

139. Espinosa N, Rothenfluh DA, Beck M, Ganz R, Leunig M: Treatment of femoro-acetabular impingement: preliminary results of labral refixation. *J Bone Joint Surg Am* 2006;88(5):925-935.

140. Clohisy JC, Nunley RM, Curry MC, Schoenecker PL: Periacetabular osteotomy for the treatment of acetabular dysplasia associated with major aspherical femoral head deformities. *J Bone Joint Surg Am* 2007;89(7):1417-1423.

CHAPTER 3

DEVELOPMENTAL DYSPLASIA OF THE HIP

MARTIN J. MORRISON III, MD
NORMAN A. JOHANSON, MD

INTRODUCTION

Developmental dysplasia of the hip (DDH) is not a single pathologic entity but rather a spectrum of disease that encompasses pathology ranging from a shallow acetabulum to a frank dislocation of the femoral head with complete absence of the acetabulum. Formerly termed congenital dislocation of the hip, the range of pathology with which it is associated is better described as DDH.[1] Not only can DDH be present at birth, it also can be the result of a disruption in the normal development and formation of the hip joint.[2] Early detection and intervention are the most important factors in the successful treatment of DDH.[3] DDH that is undiagnosed or untreated in childhood has a different presentation and symptoms in adulthood and will require more complicated treatment interventions. Total hip arthroplasty (THA), discussed later in this chapter, has become the treatment of choice in adults with symptomatic DDH.[5-10]

Formation of a normal hip joint requires balanced growth between a spherical femoral head that is concentrically reduced in a developing acetabulum.[11-14] DDH may be the end product of multiple etiologies that alter this intimate relationship.[15-18] Alterations in the shape of the femoral head and/or the acetabulum result in joint incongruence with abnormal intra-articular pressures and a range of hip pathology[19]

It is important to distinguish DDH in the otherwise healthy individual from the variations of DDH that occur in neuromuscular conditions, such as cerebral palsy and myelomeningocele, and in association with syndromes, such as Larsen syndrome or arthrogryposis. Teratologic hip dislocations occur in utero and have various etiologies as well as different treatment indications and outcomes when compared with DDH in the healthy individual, and are not discussed in this chapter.

PEDIATRIC SEQUELAE
Incidence

One in 1,000 children is born with hip dislocation, and 10 in 1,000 have lesser degrees of hip pathology that are included in the diagnosis of DDH.[12,14] Varied incidence of DDH has been reported on the basis of race, ethnicity, and geography, ranging from as high as 67 per 1,000 live births in Native Americans[20] to a near absence of the disease in African populations.[21] Infants who are swaddled tightly with their hips in extension, adduction, and internal rotation are at greater risk for hip instability and dysplasia. Cultures that care for infants by positioning their hips in the safe position (that is, in flexion, abduction, and external rotation) have a relatively low incidence of DDH. Independent risk factors such as being a firstborn child, breech position in utero, female sex, multiple gestation, oligohydramnios, and a family

Neither Dr. Morrison nor any immediate family member has received anything of value from or has stock or stock options held in a commercial company or institution related directly or indirectly to the subject of this chapter. Dr. Johanson or an immediate family member has received royalties from Exactech, and serves as a board member, owner, officer, or committee member of the American Academy of Orthopaedic Surgeons.

history of DDH are associated with an increased risk of DDH.[12,14] Metatarsus adductus, deformities of the lower extremities, congenital dislocation of the knee, congenital muscular torticollis, and generalized ligamentous laxity are reported to have lesser degrees of association with DDH.[12,14]

Evaluation

If DDH is not diagnosed and treated early, secondary soft-tissue changes, including contracture of the iliopsoas tendon and the transverse acetabular ligament with distortion of the limbus[22] and hypertrophied ligamentum teres femoris, will impede concentric and stable reduction of the hip joint.[16-18,23]

Physical Examination

A diagnosis of hip instability in the newborn during the first year of life is made by careful clinical examination of the relaxed child. The Ortolani and Barlow maneuvers as well as specific hip range-of-motion testing in the undiapered child are the mainstays of examination. After 3 months of age, soft-tissue contracture prohibits gross instability that could be observed earlier in life by performing the Ortolani or Barlow maneuver. Asymmetric hip abduction, limb-length discrepancy (LLD), and hip abduction less than 45° for each hip (in bilateral hip instability) become more reliable clinical signs of DDH as the child ages.

Imaging

In the presence of a dislocated or dislocatable hip, or with irreducible hip dislocation in the newborn (teratologic hip dislocation), radiographs of the hips and pelvis should be obtained to rule out other coexisting pathology. Lesser degrees of hip instability, such as the subluxatable hip, are more difficult to diagnose clinically and radiographically. Dynamic ultrasonography helps document mild degrees of hip instability and acetabular dysplasia. Immaturity of the acetabulum in the newborn may frequently be interpreted as dysplasia. In a stable hip, the acetabulum will develop normally without intervention. Hip ultrasonography is also useful[24,25] in the infant treated with a Pavlik harness because the relationship between the nonossified cartilage of the femoral head and the acetabulum may be clearly seen with the harness in place.[26]

Commonly Used Childhood Interventions

Early detection of hip instability in the infant allows successful and safe reduction of the hip[27,28] with use of the Pavlik harness. Abduction orthoses are also used to reduce and to stabilize the unstable hip; however, the Pavlik harness is preferable because it provides a stable safe zone based on flexion of the hip and limitation of hip adduction. Placing the hip in abduction to foster reduction of the joint is associated with the development of osteonecrosis. Appropriate use and positioning of the Pavlik harness avoids fixed abduction and allows a free range of motion of the hip within the confines of the harness. The complications reported with the Pavlik harness used for treatment of DDH have universally been associated with improper application of the harness. These complications include the inability to reduce DDH, osteonecrosis (when the harness is used as a forced abduction device),[29] fixed dislocation of the unstable hip, and femoral neurapraxia with excessive flexion of the anterior Pavlik straps.

In children older than 12 months or those who have an unstable hip that remains irreducible, closed reduction under anesthesia and hip spica casting or surgical reduction and stabilization may be required. In children up to 6 years of age, surgical reduction of the hip joint usually requires femoral shortening and a pelvic osteotomy to resolve severe acetabular dysplasia.[30,31]

Outcomes

When DDH is not diagnosed or goes untreated early in life, patients demonstrate progressive pathology and symptoms develop by the fifth decade. Advanced acetabular dysplasia, increasing instability, and osteoarthritis of the hip joint[32-34] may result in a significant LLD, a Trendelenburg gait, severe limitation of hip motion (especially in internal rotation), or an antalgic gait. A significant negative effect is noted in the adult with DDH, with decreasing function and increasing discomfort.[35,36]

When patients with DDH are treated in infancy or early childhood, a 90% success rate is expected.[37] If osteonecrosis occurs as the result of treatment, long-term results are not favorable and later interventions may be required.

ADULT SEQUELAE

Age at presentation for the evaluation of symptoms of DDH is influenced by multiple factors including grade of dysplasia, bilaterality, sex, and degree of secondary arthritis. Patients with DDH are treated with THA at a mean age of 50 years (range, 16 to 80 years).

Presenting Symptoms

Lower grades of hip dysplasia are associated with later development of symptoms and functional impairment. Dysplasia that concentrates maximal forces at the lateral weight-bearing surface of the acetabulum (Crowe types II and III; Hartofilakidis type II) is associated with the highest risk of premature secondary arthritic changes in the hip.[16-18] As subluxation progresses to dislocation, the acetabular labrum bears a higher proportion of load through the joint and may slow the development of early degenerative arthritis. The labrum will ultimately fail, however, resulting in degenerative arthritis. Hip joint pain and joint-related pain may occur in patients with hip dysplasia without significant joint space narrowing. The surgeon must then weigh the benefits of THA versus osteotomy. THA will more rapidly and reliably restore hip stability and relieve pain, but it involves the premature removal of viable hyaline cartilage, which might be preserved by using a femoral or periacetabular osteotomy.[38-41]

Unilateral Versus Bilateral DDH

Bilateral DDH may be missed in childhood because asymmetry is not observed during physical examination of the hip. Bilateral DDH is well tolerated for many decades and does not become symptomatic until later in life. Patients with unilateral DDH are more likely to seek evaluation and treatment earlier than those with bilateral DDH because of functional impairment secondary to a significant LLD (**Figure 1**). This situation is most commonly observed in patients with unilateral high hip dislocation (Crowe type IV or Hartofilakidis type III).

A significant LLD may contribute to the development of low back pain or knee pain, compensatory lumbar scoliosis, or valgus knee deformity secondary to hypoplasia of the lateral femoral condyle. In the young patient, apparent spinal deformity is supple and usually resolves with restoration of equal leg lengths. In the older patient, however, the spinal deformity is more rigid and does not resolve, so spinopelvic imbalance may result with limb equalization.

Secondary Degenerative Arthritis

Secondary degenerative arthritis of the hip associated with DDH is the result of joint instability and increased load concentration in the superolateral edge of the acetabulum. Inherently abnormal early development of the hip combined with coexisting adverse effects of treatment, such as osteonecrosis and persistent joint incongruity, are associated with degenerative changes at long-term follow-up.

Evaluation

It is important to have an understanding of the intensity and location of the patient's pain. Groin pain at rest or related to activity is the most common presenting symptom; however, pain also may be experienced posteriorly with radiation to the low back and the posterior thigh. Posterior thigh pain that radiates distal to the knee should increase suspicion for radiculopathy. Calf pain also may occur because of chronic irritation of the gastrocnemius-soleus complex secondary to arthritic changes in the knee.

History

A detailed assessment of the patient's functional impairment and desired activity level is important in determining the appropriateness of treatment with THA. Younger patients with unilateral hip dislocation, a significant LLD, and coexisting knee and/or spine involvement present earlier for evaluation and treatment recommendations. The young, healthy patient who has no pain at rest may engage in physical activities that precipitate symptoms or may express a strong desire to be "normal" and able to resume all vigorous physical activities. Careful, accurate assessment of the relationship of the patient's symptoms to the degree of functional impairment as well as clearly defined expectations of surgical intervention may require multiple examinations of the patient over several months.

Physical Examination

The physical examination of the patient with DDH is highly dependent on the patient's age, stage of DDH, and presence of degenerative arthritis of the hip. The spectrum of DDH ranges from the older patient with mild bilateral hip dysplasia with advanced arthritis to the young patient with a unilateral high hip dislocation.

FIGURE 1

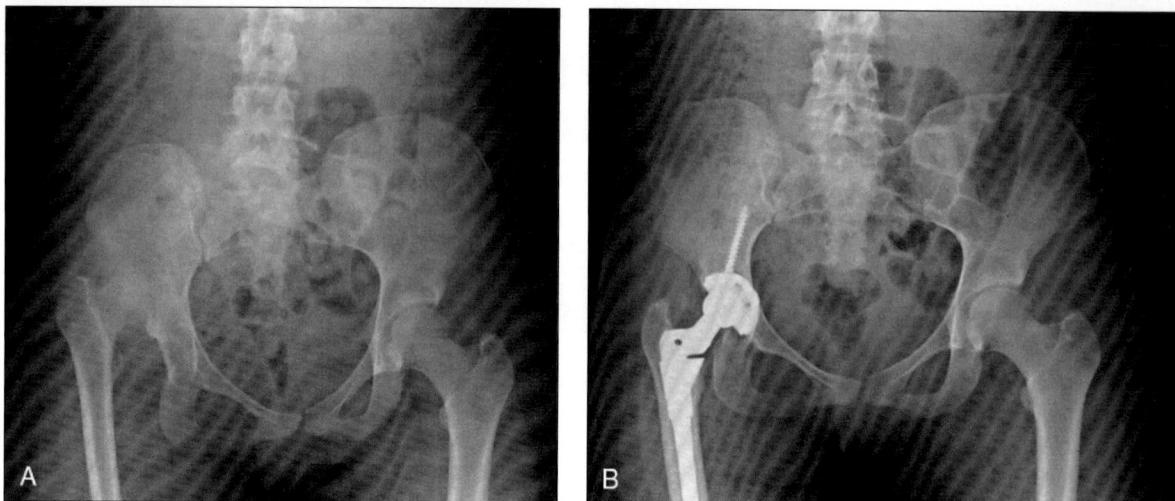

AP radiographs of the pelvis of a 17-year-old girl with a Crowe type IV hip who underwent total hip arthroplasty. **A,** Preoperative AP view. **B,** Postoperative AP view illustrates the restoration of the hip center and the reduction of the limb-length discrepancy.

The patient with unilateral high hip dislocation will stand with the ipsilateral foot in equinus to balance the pelvis. The coexistence of flexion and adduction contractures of the dislocated hip with valgus deformity of the knee exaggerates the apparent LLD and complicates preoperative planning. Valgus deformity of the knee is observed with unilateral high hip dislocation and may be associated with significant ligamentous laxity of the knee joint that may adversely affect rehabilitation after THA or progressively degenerate and require surgical intervention.

Hyperlordosis of the lumbar spine or fixed lumbar scoliosis will also influence the evaluation of LLD and are important considerations in the decision to restore limb equality. Equalization of limb lengths in the face of fixed lumbar scoliosis could result in lateral decompensation of the trunk toward the patient's unaffected limb. This uncovers the pelvis on the affected side and creates the false impression of an LLD, with the affected side now appearing longer than the unaffected side. Assessment of the patient's posture and comfort level while the affected lower limb is supported by leveling blocks helps with decision making and avoiding complications.

At physical examination, distinguishing between hip disease with or without a spinal disorder and radiculop-athy may be prohibited by the profound loss of hip joint motion. When an adequate neurologic examination cannot be performed because of severely limited hip motion, a more specific neurologic consultation with imaging of the lumbosacral spine may be indicated.

The physical examination of the patient with unilateral or bilateral low-grade degenerative arthritis of the hip is similar to the examination of the patient with osteoarthritis of the hip. In this patient population, the LLD rarely exceeds 2 cm, and valgus deformity of the knee is not common; however, secondary contractures of the hip in flexion and adduction may influence the assessment. Because the degree of degenerative arthritis determines the severity of lost motion, end-stage arthritis of both hips results in severe loss of abduction and significant functional impairment. Secondary lumbar spine or ipsilateral knee problems may develop from compensatory abnormal forces that are chronically delivered to these areas.

Imaging Studies

Weight-bearing AP radiographs of the hips and pelvis combined with supine AP and lateral views of each hip allow assessment of the grade of dysplasia and the degree of degenerative arthritis. An LLD may be estimated by comparing the difference between the distances of the lesser trochanter of each femur from a horizontal line that passes either through the tips of the ischial tuberosities or from the inferiormost extent of the acetabular teardrops. With a significant LLD, full-length orthoroentgenograms can be obtained to ascertain the true LLD. A CT scan of the pelvis and hips[24] provides information regarding the integrity of the anterior and posterior acetabular walls, the medial and superior acetabular bone stock,[42] and the relationship between the femoral shaft and neck in patients with high-grade DDH and secondary anatomic abnormalities of the hip and pelvis. Increased femoral anteversion is commonly associated with DDH[43,44] and may be determined preoperatively. Because marked differences in femoral shaft morphology and canal diameters less than 9 mm have been observed in DDH, CT scans facilitate preoperative planning and implant selection by accurately measuring the width of the canal.

Interventions for the Adult Patient

Although published reports of outcomes in patients with severe DDH treated using THA are favorable, these studies have originated from centers with extensive experience in performing THA for severe DDH.[9,10,45-52] THA performed in the patient with high-grade DDH by a surgeon inexperienced with this procedure and with the implants used in routine THA for osteoarthritis of the hip has a significant risk of less-than-favorable results. Early revision surgery[53] to treat prosthetic dislocation or loss of implant fixation is possible.

When undetected or even mild DDH persists into adulthood, the mainstay of treatment is THA.[5,45] DDH represents a wide spectrum of disease, and results can be difficult to interpret. When performing THA, the surgical management and technical difficulties encountered vary greatly between patients with minimal hip dysplasia and those with highly dysmorphic pathoanatomy. Crowe et al[54] (**Table 1**) and Hartofilakidis et al[55] (**Table 2**) have proposed classification systems to correlate the staging of pathology with anticipated technical difficulties. A new classification system proposed by Gaston et al[56] (**Table 3**) categorizes changes in both the acetabulum and femur independently and includes postsurgical changes of the acetabulum and femur with or without the presence of hardware.

TABLE 1 Crowe Classification of Adult DDH

Type	Hip Subluxation
I	<50%
II	50%–75%
III	75%–100%
IV	100%

Data adapted from Crowe JF, Mani VJ, Ranawat CS: Total hip replacement in congenital dislocation and dysplasia of the hip. *J Bone Joint Surg Am* 1979;61(1):15-23.

The decision to proceed with THA in the patient with an advanced stage of DDH is determined on the basis of the surgeon's experience in concert with the patient's grade of dysplasia, severity of arthritic change, level of pain, and functional impairment. A thorough discussion of the risks and benefits of THA allows the patient to clearly express values, concerns, preferences, and expectations regarding THA and to fully participate in the decision-making process. The usual risks of complications with THA are increased in patients with DDH because of diminished acetabular and femoral size, deficient bone stock, alterations in acetabular and femoral version, and LLD. Previous surgeries about the acetabulum and proximal femur may compound difficulties in performing THA in patients with DDH.[57]

Hip Subluxation and Acetabular Dysplasia

Patients with low-grade DDH may be treated in most situations with primary cemented or cementless implants with nonmodular femoral stems, even in the presence of severe degenerative arthritis. As subluxation and acetabular dysplasia increase, medialization of the acetabulum is more likely to be required[58] to return the center of rotation of the hip to a more normal location (**Figure 2**). The resulting laxity of soft tissue should be addressed either with a lateralized femoral stem or a lateralized acetabular liner. An increase in native anteversion of the femoral neck is improved by using a cemented femoral stem or modular stem, which allows relative retroversion of the prosthesis in relation to the femoral

TABLE 2 Hartofilakidis Classification of Congenital Hip Disease in Adults

Type	Acetabular Findings
I (dysplasia)	Superior segmental deficiency, shallow due to osteophytes
II (low dislocation)	Anterior and posterior segmental deficiency, narrow opening, inadequate depth, increased anteversion, lack of posterior bone stock
III (high dislocation)	Segmental deficiency of entire rim, narrow rim, inadequate depth, excessive anteversion, abnormal distribution of bone stock (primarily superoposteriorly)

Data adapted from Hartofilakidis G, Stamos K, Karachalios T, Ioannidis TT, Zacharakis N: Congenital hip disease in adults: Classification of acetabular deficiencies and operative treatment with acetabuloplasty combined with total hip arthroplasty. *J Bone Joint Surg Am* 1996;78(5):683-692.

TABLE 3 Gaston Classification for Adult DDH

Location and Type	Findings
Acetabulum	
AI	Dysplastic
AII	Low dislocation
AIII	Postsurgical
AIIIa	With hardware
AIIIb	Without hardware
Femur	
FI	Dysplastic
FII	High dislocation
FIII	Postsurgical
FIIIa	With hardware
FIIIb	Without hardware

Data adapted from Gaston MS, Gaston P, Donaldson P, Howie CR: A new classification system for the adult dysplastic hip requiring total hip arthroplasty: A reliability study. *Hip Int* 2009;19(2):96-101.

neck and restores stability at the prosthetic joint couple. Reducing the anteversion of the acetabular component also ameliorates component mismatch.

Severe Acetabular Dysplasia and Femoral Anteversion

When severe deficiency exists in the anterior acetabular wall, anteversion of the acetabular component is increased to obtain adequate bone coverage, and retroversion of the femoral neck in excess of 45° may be needed. Under these conditions, it is unlikely that a cemented femoral stem of adequate size could be effective; a modular femoral stem would be a better solution to this problem. For the patient with a femoral canal diameter greater than 9 mm, several modular femoral stems exist that would facilitate appropriate adjustment of the femoral neck version, length, and offset. Few options exist when the femoral canal diameter is less than 9 mm. A monoblock stem is needed for the very small femoral canal, either in the form of a custom-manufactured implant or a modular off-the-shelf implant, which permits maximum flexibility of neck version, achieves distal fit and rotational stability, and integrates with a conical metaphyseal sleeve for proximal support. The metaphyseal sleeve has an extension that is milled to size and fits inside the remnant of the femoral neck. If an osteotomy is performed below the femoral neck or no remnant of a femoral neck exists, a purely conical sleeve may be used.

FIGURE 2

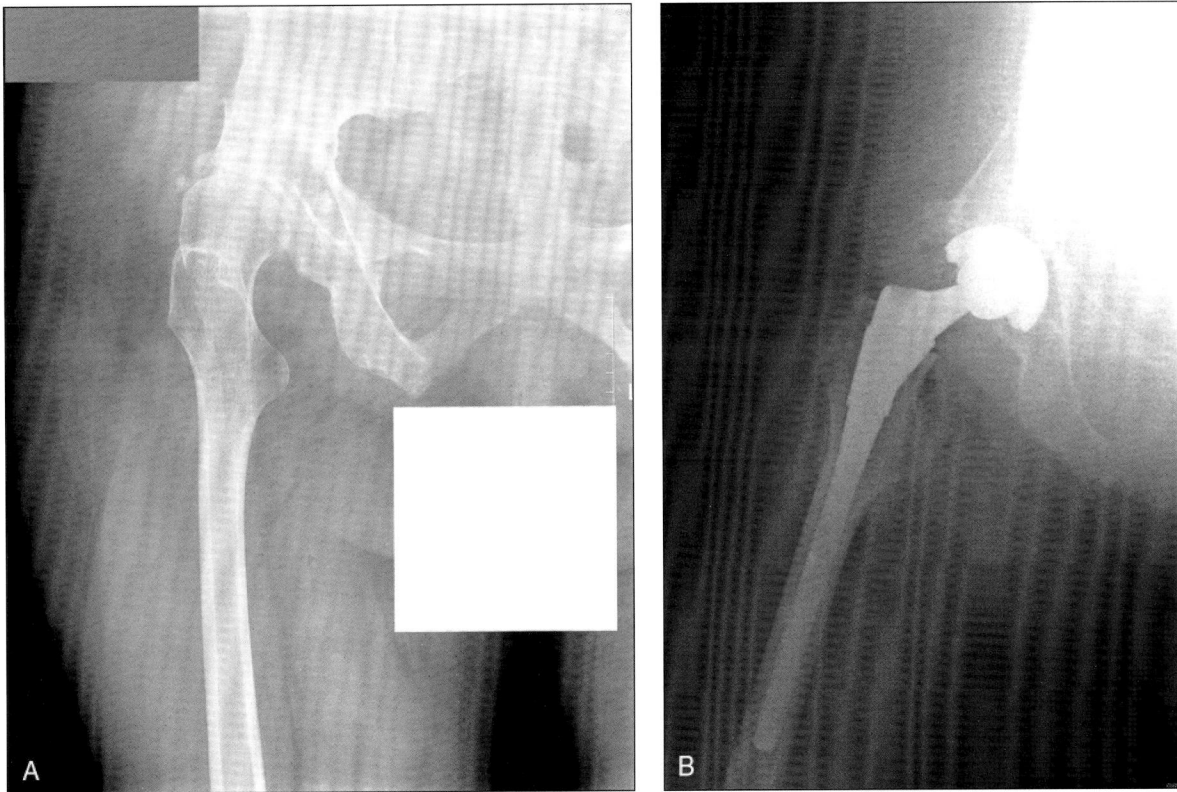

AP radiographs of the hip of a 39-year-old woman who underwent bilateral triple innominate osteotomy at 9 years of age. **A,** Radiograph obtained before total hip arthroplasty (THA). **B,** Radiograph obtained after THA demonstrates medialization of the acetabulum to restore the center of rotation.

High Hip Dislocation

The surgeon faces significant reconstruction challenges when treating a high hip dislocation. These challenges include (1) a deformed atrophic femoral head and neck that articulates with fibrous tissue that blends into the lateral surface of the iliac wing (false acetabulum); (2) fibrous encapsulation of the hip joint with varying degrees of laxity; (3) atrophic and contracted abductor mechanism with fibrosis and fatty degeneration; and (4) a rudimentary true acetabulum that is small, shallow, and poorly defined.

Achieving the surgical objectives requires successful completion of the following critical steps: (1) capsulotomy or capsulectomy and mobilization of the femoral head; (2) executing the femoral neck osteotomy at the appropriate level; (3) exposing and reaming the acetabulum to the appropriate size and location of the hip center; (4) pericapsular soft-tissue release to achieve reduction of the reconstructed hip; and (5) decision for and execution of femoral shortening osteotomy and femoral reaming.

In a high hip dislocation, capsular structures are attenuated and blend with periarticular fibroadipose tissue. Dense scar tissue may be encountered anteriorly and anterolaterally in previously operated hips. Pediatric hip procedures are most commonly performed through anterior approaches and leave posterior tissues intact without scar formation. In previously operated hips, anterior fibrous adhesions to the femoral head may increase the difficulty of mobilizing the proximal femur.

In addition to postoperative scarring, the superior capsule of the dislocated hip is frequently hypertrophied because of the chronic stress of weight bearing placed on the overlying soft tissues by the dislocated femoral head. In view of significant soft-tissue resistance, application of excessive torque that may result in fracture of the femur should be avoided.

Femoral Neck Osteotomy

Femoral neck osteotomy and removal of the femoral head facilitate resection of the capsule from the posterior femoral neck and aid in locating the posterior wall of the true acetabulum. In a high hip dislocation, normal anatomic landmarks that differentiate among the femoral head, femoral neck, and greater trochanter may be severely distorted. The configuration of the osteotomy depends on the choice of femoral implant. For a conventional femoral stem, an oblique osteotomy should be performed, with attention given to the angle of femoral neck version. For commonly used modular stems, the femoral neck osteotomy is made transverse to the axis of the shaft, passes lateral to the trochanteric ridge, and proximally parallels the sagittal orientation of the greater trochanter. In the case of severe proximal femoral deformity, the greater trochanter may be hypoplastic and located more posteriorly than normal. When the femoral neck osteotomy is performed more distally to moderate the effect of soft-tissue tightness and the resistance to moving the hip center of rotation distally, a greater risk of fracture of the greater trochanter exists.

Acetabular Exposure and Reaming

Locating the true acetabulum in a high hip dislocation requires extensive débridement of fibroadipose tissue that extends inferiorly into the acetabular fossa. Prior to reaming, the inferomedial extent of the acetabulum and the anatomic location of the radiographic teardrop should be identified, as well as the anterior, posterior, and superior acetabular rims. Because of vascular hypertrophy, this step may be associated with significant bleeding.

Preoperative CT evaluation of bone stock is critical to successful reaming of the acetabulum.[59] Reaming begins with a small reamer (30 to 34 mm) that is directed medially and posteriorly to better define the location and extent of possible bone coverage. Careful, sequen-

tial reaming enlarges the acetabular margins and more precisely localizes the height of the hip center of rotation. The superior margin of the acetabulum is identified by reaming the sclerotic plate of bone that partially covers the true acetabulum and represents the superiormost position for the acetabulum without the use of structural augmentation. The sclerotic plate of bone converges with the outer table of the ilium and will disappear quickly with overreaming. Successful acetabular reaming depends on the integration of medialization and enlargement that optimizes stability and host bone contact with the cementless acetabular component. Stability may be augmented by passing fixation screws superiorly between the two tables of the ilium or into the ischium. The flexibility to adjust femoral neck version that is possible with use of the modular femoral stem allows optimal acetabular–host bone contact and structural support.

Distal Displacement of the Proximal Femur

After setting the acetabular position, full mobilization of the proximal femur is accomplished by releasing all capsular attachments to the femur, stripping the abductors from the ilium, releasing the iliopsoas, and transecting the iliotibial band. The combination of a modestly superior placement of the acetabular center ($\leq$1.5 cm) and distal placement of the center of the femoral head may be necessary to achieve reduction of the hip joint.

The acceptable range of acetabular position in the correction of high hip dislocation is controversial. An acetabular position with a high hip center has been associated with an increase in prosthetic loosening.[60] However, returning the acetabular component to its native position may result in excessive soft-tissue release, lengthening the limb to a degree that requires a femoral shortening osteotomy, a structural allograft to maintain position, or sacrifice of adequate host bone for long-term fixation. When necessary, reaming the acetabulum superiorly to maximize host bone support and to facilitate reduction of the hip may be prudent.[7] The surgeon's experience and judgment regarding multiple factors that may influence outcome are of primary importance.

Placing the femoral component more distal along the femoral canal is limited by the risk of greater trochanteric impingement of the posterior rim of the acetabulum or the acetabular component. In addition, with a more distal femoral neck osteotomy, loss of the internal contour of the femoral neck may compromise rotational stability of the femoral component. This loss may be compensated for by using a fully porous coated implant or a fluted femoral stem. Modular femoral stems have conical metaphyseal components that accommodate anatomic variations.

Femoral Shortening

The indications for a femoral shortening osteotomy in patients with high hip dislocation have not been standardized, and multiple factors influence the surgeon's decision to perform femoral shortening osteotomy.[61-64] These factors include anticipating the optimal net lengthening based on the preoperative superior displacement of the femoral head, the expected acetabular position, and the cumulative effect of elongation on the sciatic nerve. Edwards et al[65] reported injury to either the peroneal division of the sciatic nerve or the sciatic nerve proper, with lengthening of 1.9 to 5.1 cm. Nagoya et al[66] reported the results of THA in 20 patients with high hip dislocation with a net lengthening up to 5.1 cm and no evidence of nerve injury. Partial to complete resolution of postoperative neurologic deficit has been reported in most patients with reported neurologic injuries following THA.[67] An evidence-based algorithm for this procedure is difficult to develop because of the relatively low occurrence of high hip dislocation secondary to DDH and the low incidence of reported nerve injury. Other complications associated with femoral shortening osteotomy include femoral fracture, component loosening, nonunion, and even nerve injury.

CONCLUSION

THA is performed to treat DDH in a younger population with a varied severity of symptoms and functional impairment. THA is associated with significant technical challenges because of the diverse pathoanatomy in this population.[68] A high degree of technical ability, experience with the uncommon problem of high hip dislocation, and critical evaluation of clinical and anatomic factors are necessary for successful outcomes of THA in this population. However, controversy exists regarding the acceptable range of position of the acetabular component, the management of the distal displacement of the proximal femur, the femoral component design and

positioning, and the maximum allowable net lengthening of the limb.[69]

REFERENCES

1. Klisic PJ: Congenital dislocation of the hip—a misleading term: Brief report. *J Bone Joint Surg Br* 1989;71(1):136.
2. Weinstein SL, Ponseti IV: Congenital dislocation of the hip. *J Bone Joint Surg Am* 1979;61(1):119-124.
3. Barlow TG: Early diagnosis and treatment of congenital dislocation of the hip. *J Bone Joint Surg Am* 1962;44:292-301.
4. Harris WH: Etiology of osteoarthritis of the hip. *Clin Orthop Relat Res* 1986(213):20-33.
5. Anderson MJ, Harris WH: Total hip arthroplasty with insertion of the acetabular component without cement in hips with total congenital dislocation or marked congenital dysplasia. *J Bone Joint Surg Am* 1999;81(3):347-354.
6. Biant LC, Bruce WJ, Assini JB, Walker PM, Walsh WR: Primary total hip arthroplasty in severe developmental dysplasia of the hip: Ten-year results using a cementless modular stem. *J Arthroplasty* 2009;24(1):27-32.
7. Erdemli B, Yilmaz C, Atalar H, Güzel B, Cetin I: Total hip arthroplasty in developmental high dislocation of the hip. *J Arthroplasty* 2005;20(8):1021-1028.
8. Hartofilakidis G, Karachalios T: Total hip arthroplasty for congenital hip disease. *J Bone Joint Surg Am* 2004;86-A(2):242-250.
9. Papachristou G, Hatzigrigoris P, Panousis K, et al: Total hip arthroplasty for developmental hip dysplasia. *Int Orthop* 2006;30(1):21-25.
10. Sochart DH, Porter ML: The long-term results of Charnley low-friction arthroplasty in young patients who have congenital dislocation, degenerative osteoarthrosis, or rheumatoid arthritis. *J Bone Joint Surg Am* 1997;79(11):1599-1617.
11. Aronsson DD, Goldberg MJ, Kling TF Jr, Roy DR: Developmental dysplasia of the hip. *Pediatrics* 1994;94(2 Pt 1):201-208.
12. Guille JT, Pizzutillo PD, MacEwen GD: Development dysplasia of the hip from birth to six months. *J Am Acad Orthop Surg* 2000;8(4):232-242.
13. Morrissy RT, Weinstein SL: Developmental Hip Dysplasia and Dislocation, in *Lovell and Winter's Pediatric Orthopaedics*, ed 6. Philadelphia, PA, Lippincott Williams & Wilkins, 2008, pp 987-1038.

14. Vitale MG, Skaggs DL: Developmental dysplasia of the hip from six months to four years of age. *J Am Acad Orthop Surg* 2001;9(6):401-411.

15. Dunn PM: Perinatal observations on the etiology of congenital dislocation of the hip. *Clin Orthop Relat Res* 1976(119):11-22.

16. Wedge JH, Wasylenko MJ: The natural history of congenital disease of the hip. *J Bone Joint Surg Br* 1979; 61-B(3):334-338.

17. Weinstein SL: Natural history and treatment outcomes of childhood hip disorders. *Clin Orthop Relat Res* 1997(344):227-242.

18. Weinstein SL: Natural history of congenital hip dislocation (CDH) and hip dysplasia. *Clin Orthop Relat Res* 1987(225):62-76.

19. Harris NH: Acetabular growth potential in congenital dislocation of the hip and some factors upon which it may depend. *Clin Orthop Relat Res* 1976(119):99-106.

20. Coleman SS: Congenital dysplasia of the hip in the Navajo infant. *Clin Orthop Relat Res* 1968(56):179-193.

21. Skirving AP, Scadden WJ: The African neonatal hip and its immunity from congenital dislocation. *J Bone Joint Surg Br* 1979;61-B(3):339-341.

22. Landa J, Benke M, Feldman DS: The limbus and the neolimbus in developmental dysplasia of the hip. *Clin Orthop Relat Res* 2008;466(4):776-781.

23. Ilfeld FW, Westin GW, Makin M: Missed or developmental dislocation of the hip. *Clin Orthop Relat Res* 1986(203):276-281.

24. Harcke HT: Imaging in congenital dislocation and dysplasia of the hip. *Clin Orthop Relat Res* 1992(281): 22-28.

25. Harcke HT, Kumar SJ: The role of ultrasound in the diagnosis and management of congenital dislocation and dysplasia of the hip. *J Bone Joint Surg Am* 1991;73(4):622-628.

26. White KK, Sucato DJ, Agrawal S, Browne R: Ultrasonographic findings in hips with a positive Ortolani sign and their relationship to Pavlik harness failure. *J Bone Joint Surg Am* 2010;92(1):113-120.

27. Ishii Y, Ponseti IV: Long-term results of closed reduction of complete congenital dislocation of the hip in children under one year of age. *Clin Orthop Relat Res* 1978(137):167-174.

28. Malvitz TA, Weinstein SL: Closed reduction for congenital dysplasia of the hip: Functional and radiographic results after an average of thirty years. *J Bone Joint Surg Am* 1994;76(12):1777-1792.

29. Cooperman DR, Wallensten R, Stulberg SD: Post-reduction avascular necrosis in congenital dislocation of the hip. *J Bone Joint Surg Am* 1980;62(2):247-258.

30. Klisić P, Janković L, Basara V: Long-term results of combined operative reduction of the hip in older children. *J Pediatr Orthop* 1988;8(5):532-534.

31. Zionts LE, MacEwen GD: Treatment of congenital dislocation of the hip in children between the ages of one and three years. *J Bone Joint Surg Am* 1986;68(6): 829-846.

32. Murray RO: The aetiology of primary osteoarthritis of the hip. *Br J Radiol* 1965;38(455):810-824.

33. Solomon L: Patterns of osteoarthritis of the hip. *J Bone Joint Surg Br* 1976;58(2):176-183.

34. Stulberg SD, Harris WH: Acetabular dysplasia and development of osteoarthritis of the hip, in Harris WH, ed: *The Hip: Proceedings of the Second Open Scientific Meeting of the Hip Society*. St Louis, MO, CV Mosby, 1974, pp 82-93.

35. Romanò CL, Frigo C, Randelli G, Pedotti A: Analysis of the gait of adults who had residua of congenital dysplasia of the hip. *J Bone Joint Surg Am* 1996;78(10): 1468-1479.

36. Tellini A, Ciccone V, Blonna D, Rossi R, Marmotti A, Castoldi F: Quality of life evaluation in patients affected by osteoarthritis secondary to congenital hip dysplasia after total hip replacement. *J Orthop Traumatol* 2008;9(3):155-158.

37. Cashman JP, Round J, Taylor G, Clarke NM: The natural history of developmental dysplasia of the hip after early supervised treatment in the Pavlik harness: A prospective, longitudinal follow-up. *J Bone Joint Surg Br* 2002;84(3):418-425.

38. Hopf A: Hüftpfannenverlagerung durch doppelte Beckenosteotomie zur Behandlung der Hüftgelenksdysplasie und Subluxation bei Jugendlichen und Erwachsenen. *Z Orthop Ihre Grenzgeb* 1966;101(4):559-586.

39. Janssen D, Kalchschmidt K, Katthagen BD: Triple pelvic osteotomy as treatment for osteoarthritis secondary to developmental dysplasia of the hip. *Int Orthop* 2009;33(6):1555-1559.

40. Millis MB, Poss R, Murphy SB: Osteotomies of the hip in the prevention and treatment of osteoarthritis. *Instr Course Lect* 1992;41:145-154.

41. Troelsen A: Surgical advances in periacetabular oste-otomy for treatment of hip dysplasia in adults. *Acta Orthop Suppl* 2009;80(332):1-33.

42. Lee BP, Cabanela ME, Wallrichs SL, Ilstrup DM: Bone-graft augmentation for acetabular deficiencies in total hip arthroplasty: Results of long-term follow-up evaluation. *J Arthroplasty* 1997;12(5):503-510.

43. Halpern AA, Tanner J, Rinsky L: Does persistent fetal femoral anteversion contribute to osteoarthritis? A preliminary report. *Clin Orthop Relat Res* 1979;145:213-216.

44. Tönnis D, Heinecke A: Acetabular and femoral antever-sion: Relationship with osteoarthritis of the hip. *J Bone Joint Surg Am* 1999;81(12):1747-1770.

45. Amstutz HC, Antoniades JT, Le Duff MJ: Results of metal-on-metal hybrid hip resurfacing for Crowe type-I and II developmental dysplasia. *J Bone Joint Surg Am* 2007;89(2):339-346.

46. Bruzzone M, La Russa M, Garzaro G, et al: Long-term results of cementless anatomic total hip replacement in dysplastic hips. *Chir Organi Mov* 2009;93(3):131-136.

47. Georgiades G, Babis GC, Hartofilakidis G: Charnley low-friction arthroplasty in young patients with osteo-arthritis: Outcomes at a minimum of twenty-two years. *J Bone Joint Surg Am* 2009;91(12):2846-2851.

48. Ioannidis TT, Zacharakis N, Magnissalis EA, Eliades G, Hartofilakidis G: Long-term behaviour of the Charn-ley offset-bore acetabular cup. *J Bone Joint Surg Br* 1998;80(1):48-53.

49. MacKenzie JR, Kelley SS, Johnston RC: Total hip replacement for coxarthrosis secondary to congenital dysplasia and dislocation of the hip: Long-term results. *J Bone Joint Surg Am* 1996;78(1):55-61.

50. Naal FD, Schmied M, Munzinger U, Leunig M, Hersche O: Outcome of hip resurfacing arthroplasty in patients with developmental hip dysplasia. *Clin Orthop Relat Res* 2009;467(6):1516-1521.

51. Paavilainen T, Hoikka V, Solonen KA: Cementless total replacement for severely dysplastic or dislocated hips. *J Bone Joint Surg Br* 1990;72(2):205-211.

52. Stans AA, Pagnano MW, Shaughnessy WJ, Hanssen AD: Results of total hip arthroplasty for Crowe Type III developmental hip dysplasia. *Clin Orthop Relat Res* 1998;348:149-157.

53. Tabutin J, Cambas PM: Hip arthroplasty up to the age of 30 and considerations in relation to subsequent revi-sion. *Hip Int* 2009;19(3):201-205.

54. Crowe JF, Mani VJ, Ranawat CS: Total hip replacement in congenital dislocation and dysplasia of the hip. *J Bone Joint Surg Am* 1979;61(1):15-23.

55. Hartofilakidis G, Stamos K, Karachalios T, Ioannidis TT, Zacharakis N: Congenital hip disease in adults: Classification of acetabular deficiencies and operative treatment with acetabuloplasty combined with total hip arthroplasty. *J Bone Joint Surg Am* 1996;78(5):683-692.

56. Gaston MS, Gaston P, Donaldson P, Howie CR: A new classification system for the adult dysplastic hip requir-ing total hip arthroplasty: A reliability study. *Hip Int* 2009;19(2):96-101.

57. Argenson JN, Flecher X, Parratte S, Aubaniac JM: Anat-omy of the dysplastic hip and consequences for total hip arthroplasty. *Clin Orthop Relat Res* 2007;465:40-45.

58. Dorr LD, Tawakkol S, Moorthy M, Long W, Wan Z: Medial protrusion technique for placement of a porous-coated, hemispherical acetabular component without cement in a total hip arthroplasty in patients who have acetabular dysplasia. *J Bone Joint Surg Am* 1999;81(1):83-92.

59. Stanton RP, Capecci R: Computed tomography for early evaluation of developmental dysplasia of the hip. *J Pediatr Orthop* 1992;12(6):727-730.

60. Pagnano W, Hanssen AD, Lewallen DG, Shaughnessy WJ: The effect of superior placement of the acetabular component on the rate of loosening after total hip ar-throplasty. *J Bone Joint Surg Am* 1996;78(7):1004-1014.

61. Bernasek TL, Haidukewych GJ, Gustke KA, Hill O, Lever-ing M: Total hip arthroplasty requiring subtrochanteric osteotomy for developmental hip dysplasia: 5- to 14-year results. *J Arthroplasty* 2007;22(6, Suppl 2):145-150.

62. Chareancholvanich K, Becker DA, Gustilo RB: Treatment of congenital dislocated hip by arthro-plasty with femoral shortening. *Clin Orthop Relat Res* 1999(360):127-135.

63. Krych AJ, Howard JL, Trousdale RT, Cabanela ME, Berry DJ: Total hip arthroplasty with shortening subtro-chanteric osteotomy in Crowe type-IV developmental dysplasia. *J Bone Joint Surg Am* 2009;91(9):2213-2221.

64. Reikerås O, Haaland JE, Lereim P: Femoral shortening in total hip arthroplasty for high developmental dysplasia of the hip. *Clin Orthop Relat Res* 2010;468(7):1949-1955.

65. Edwards BN, Tullos HS, Noble PC: Contributory factors and etiology of sciatic nerve palsy in total hip arthro-plasty. *Clin Orthop Relat Res* 1987;218:136-141.

66. Nagoya S, Kaya M, Sasaki M, Tateda K, Kosukegawa I, Yamashita T: Cementless total hip replacement with subtrochanteric femoral shortening for severe developmental dysplasia of the hip. *J Bone Joint Surg Br* 2009;91(9):1142-1147.

67. Lewallen DG: Neurovascular injury associated with hip arthroplasty. *Instr Course Lect* 1998;47:275-283.

68. Peters CL, Erickson JA, Anderson L, Anderson AA, Weiss J: Hip-preserving surgery: Understanding complex pathomorphology. *J Bone Joint Surg Am* 2009;91(Suppl 6):42-58.

69. Lai KA, Shen WJ, Huang LW, Chen MY: Cementless total hip arthroplasty and limb-length equalization in patients with unilateral Crowe type-IV hip dislocation. *J Bone Joint Surg Am* 2005;87(2):339-345.

CHAPTER 4

OSTEOCHONDRITIS DISSECANS OF THE KNEE, ANTERIOR CRUCIATE LIGAMENT INJURY, AND MENISCAL TEARS

JEREMY S. FRANK, MD

LYLE J. MICHELI, MD

MININDER S. KOCHER, MD, MPH

INTRODUCTION

Knee injuries in the pediatric and adolescent athlete are occurring in increased numbers with expanded participation in organized youth athletics, less free play, and increased single-sport focus at younger ages. Injury patterns are unique to the growing musculoskeletal system and specific to the demands of the involved sport. Prompt diagnosis, effective treatment, and gradual return to play are all critical factors in forestalling the potential progression to early degenerative changes. This chapter discusses three common pediatric orthopaedic knee conditions and their sequelae in the adult knee: osteochondritis dissecans (OCD), anterior cruciate ligament (ACL) injuries, and meniscal tears.

OSTEOCHONDRITIS DISSECANS

OCD is an acquired, potentially reversible idiopathic lesion of the subchondral bone that results in delamination and sequestration with or without articular cartilage involvement and instability.[1] The etiology of OCD is controversial (inflammation versus repetitive trauma versus ischemia). OCD is classified based on anatomic location, scintigraphic findings, surgical appearance, and chronologic age.[1] OCD can be further subdivided into juvenile and adult forms, depending on physeal maturity.

Most observers think that OCD only occurs in the immature skeleton, but it may manifest clinically in adolescence or early adulthood. Although exact epidemiologic

Dr. Micheli or an immediate family member has received research or institutional support from Genzyme. Dr. Kocher or an immediate family member serves as a board member, owner, officer, or committee member of the American Academy of Orthopaedic Surgeons, the ACL Study Group, the American Orthopaedic Society for Sports Medicine, the Herodicus Society, the Pediatric Orthopaedic Society of North America, and the Steadman Hawkins Research Foundation; has received royalties from Biomet; serves as a paid consultant to or is an employee of Biomet, CONMED Linvatec, Covidian, OrthoPediatrics, PediPed, Regen Biologics, and Smith & Nephew; has received research or institutional support from CONMED Linvatec; and has stock or stock options held in Pivot Medical. Neither Dr. Frank nor any immediate family member has received anything of value from or has stock or stock options held in a commercial company or institution related directly or indirectly to the subject of this chapter.

statistics are not known, Lindén[2] estimated the prevalence of OCD to be between 15 and 30 individuals per 100,000. Boys age 10 to 15 years appear to have the highest rate of incidence; however, growing participation in competitive sports by children of both sexes at younger ages has decreased the mean age of onset of OCD. Sex-based differences indicate a preponderance of male patients, with an approximate male-to-female ratio ranging from 2:1 to 3:1. Bilateral lesions have been reported in 15% to 33% of cases.[3] More than 70% of OCD lesions are typically found in the posterolateral aspect of the medial femoral condyle; OCD lesions of the lateral condyle, trochlea, and patella have been noted less often.

Early presentation often involves poorly defined symptoms including generalized knee pain, stiffness, catching, and various amounts of intermittent swelling. Without appropriate imaging (radiography and MRI), OCD lesions can worsen until a correct diagnosis is confirmed. Crawford and Safran[3] proposed a treatment algorithm for juvenile OCD (**Figure 1**). Early stable lesions can be treated with a minimum of 3 months of activity restriction, protected weight bearing, bracing, physical therapy, and NSAIDs. Unstable lesions traditionally require arthroscopic intervention using either antegrade or retrograde drilling and/or fixation.

Randomized controlled clinical trials have not been conducted for either surgical or nonsurgical treatment of OCD of the knee. However, Hefti et al[4] conducted a large multicenter review of the European Pediatric Orthopaedic Society (509 knees [318 juvenile, 191 adult] in 452 patients) that revealed several important findings: open physis, younger age, smaller lesion size, optimal lesion location (medial femoral condyle is better than patellofemoral, which is better than lateral femoral condyle), and chronicity (acute is better than chronic) were all positive predictors of healing.[4] Cahill[5] reported that 50% of nonsurgically treated juvenile OCD lesions healed within a 10- to 18-month period, provided the physis remained open and patient compliance was maintained. Wall et al[6] found that in two thirds of immature patients, 6 months of nonsurgical treatment that included activity modification and immobilization resulted in progressive healing of stable OCD lesions. Lesions with increased size and associated swelling and/or mechanical symptoms at presentation were less likely to heal. Kocher et al[7] also noted excellent functional and radiographic

outcomes with transarticular arthroscopic drilling of isolated, stable juvenile OCD lesions of the medial femoral condyle with an intact articular surface after 6 months of nonsurgical management had failed. Failure to attain healing and revascularization of the necrotic subchondral bone can result in complete lesion fragmentation, large osteochondral defects, and ultimately, early degenerative changes in the knee. Kocher et al[8] reported high healing rates, good functional outcomes, and low complication rates with internal fixation of unstable juvenile OCD lesions, even for detached lesions and in patients who have already undergone surgery for OCD.

Adult Sequelae

OCD lesions that have not revascularized by adulthood have a greater propensity for instability and typically follow a clinical course that is progressive and unremitting. Patients commonly present with reports of swelling and stiffness as well as mechanical symptoms such as locking and/or catching of the knee. These mechanical symptoms often indicate the presence of a loose, unstable fragment, which can portend a worse prognosis.

Physical examination must start with an evaluation of the patient's gait. An antalgic gait can be present with both stable and unstable lesions. Joint line and/or condylar tenderness can often be appreciated with palpation. The Wilson test is performed by extending the knee from 90°. Pain at 30° of flexion and relief with tibial external rotation is a positive sign for OCD in the femoral condyle. Conrad and Stanitski[9] demonstrated low sensitivity and a poor predictive value with this maneuver in 32 patients with radiographically proved OCD, 75% of whom had a negative result for the Wilson test. Other findings may include an effusion, crepitus with range of motion, and quadriceps atrophy.

Traditionally, diagnostic evaluation should include plain radiography and MRI. Plain radiographs are necessary to characterize and localize the OCD lesion in both children and adults, to rule out other bony injury, to evaluate skeletal maturity, and to determine the age of the lesion.[1] AP, lateral, notch, and skyline views should be included. Cahill and Berg[10] described a method of localizing lesions by dividing the knee into 15 distinct zones (**Figure 2**). Although important for research applications, this system has provided limited use in daily clinical activities.

FIGURE 1

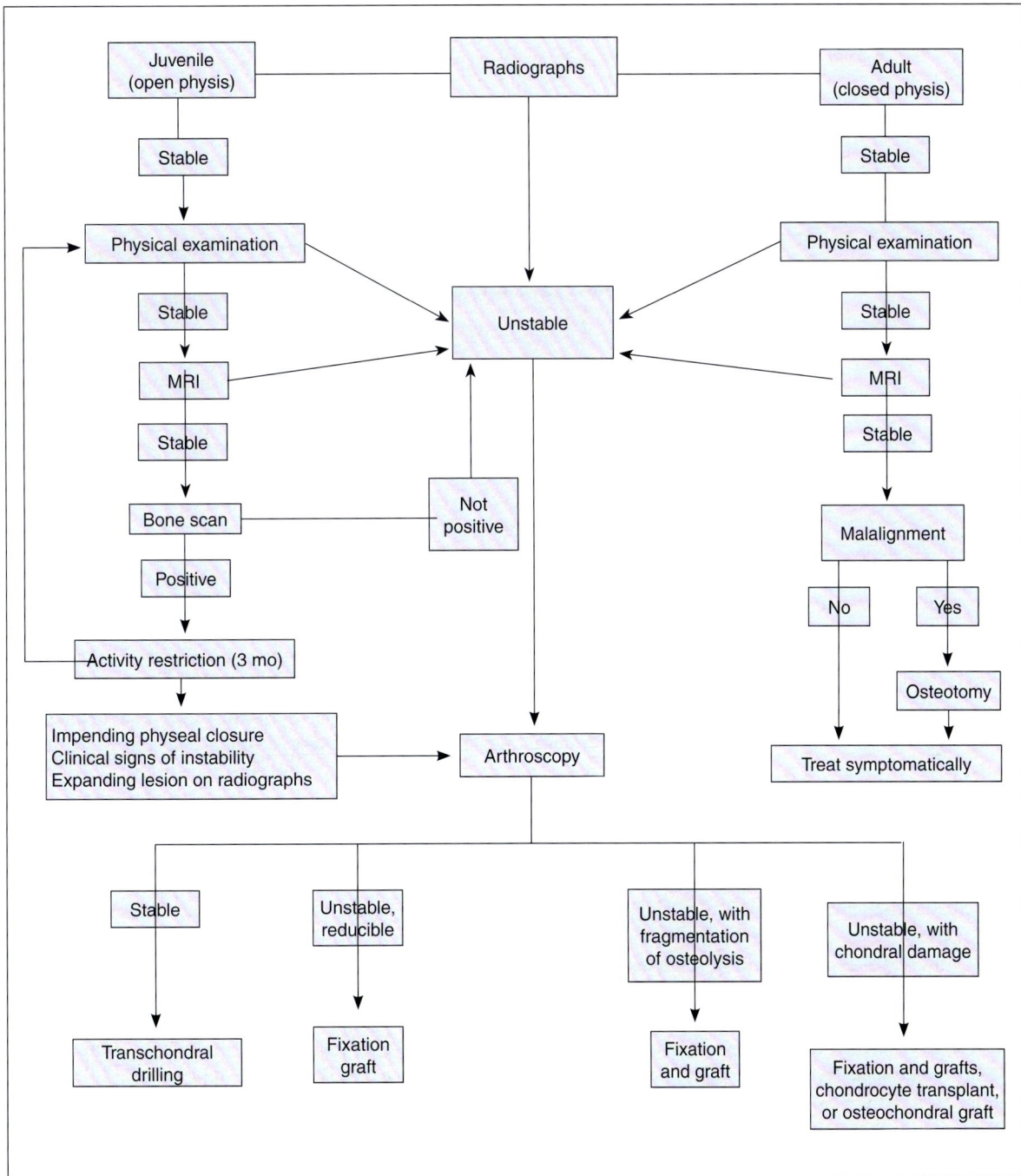

Treatment algorithm for osteochondritis dissecans of the knee. (Adapted from Crawford DC, Safran MR: Osteochondritis dissecans of the knee. *J Am Acad Orthop Surg* 2006;14[2]:90-100.)

FIGURE 2

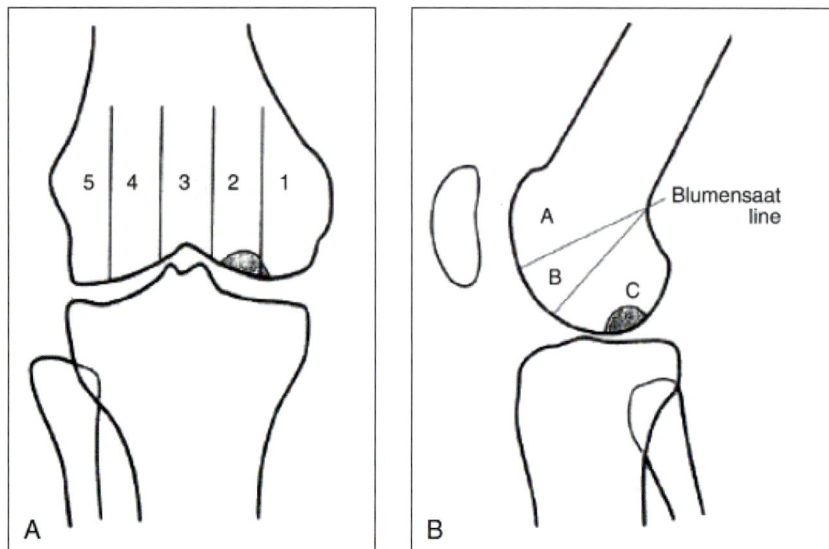

AP (**A**) and lateral (**B**) views of the knee demonstrate the 15 alphanumeric radiographic regions described by Cahill and Berg. The five numbered zones on the AP view are divided centrally by the notch (zone 3). The lettered zones on the lateral view are divided by the Blumensaat line anteriorly and the posterior cortical line. The crescent-shaped shaded area in each view of the distal femur represents an old lesion. (Adapted from Crawford DC, Safran MR: Osteochondritis dissecans of the knee. *J Am Acad Orthop Surg* 2006;14[2]:90-100.)

Nuclear imaging, most notably technetium Tc-99m bone scanning, has also been used in OCD evaluation. The bone scans can help assess both blood flow and osteoblast activity at the lesion site. Cahill et al[11] proposed a classification system based on technetium Tc-99m scintigraphic findings. The authors later reported limited correlation between this staging system and the prediction of lesion stability and/or the need for subsequent surgery.

MRI has become a routine part of the diagnostic evaluation of OCD in most treatment centers. Several studies have demonstrated its accuracy in estimating lesion size as well as the status of the cartilage and subchondral bone.[4,12,13] Moreover, MRI can identify the extent of bony edema, the appearance of a high signal intensity zone beneath the fragment, and the presence of loose bodies, which are characteristic of OCD lesions.[4] Pill et al[13] compared clinical outcomes with imaging measurements (MRI and plain radiography) and found that nonsurgical treatment failed more often in older patients with one or more signs of chondral disruption seen on MRI than in younger patients with intact cartilage margins and no signs of fragment instability.

Interventions for the Adult Patient

Compared with juvenile OCD, adult OCD typically follows a more insidious and unremitting course. As a re-sult, nonsurgical treatment in the adult is rarely successful. After physeal closure, the capacity for healing dramatically declines and the potential for eventual instability, loosening, and detachment of loose bodies is high. Therefore, early aggressive surgical management is generally indicated to maintain the articular congruency and integrity of the joint. In the rare instance of an adult with OCD whose knee is stable both on physical examination and MRI and with no malalignment, nonsurgical symptomatic treatment (weight-bearing restrictions, bracing, and NSAIDs) may be indicated.

Indications for surgical management include detached or unstable lesions noted on physical examination and diagnostic imaging as well as failure of nonsurgical treatment. Garrett[14] argued that skeletal maturity is also an absolute indication for surgical intervention. Smillie[15] argued that an open lesion, which demonstrates dissection of synovial fluid into the lesion, is also an indication for surgical treatment. Both adult and juvenile forms of OCD primarily affect subchondral bone and secondarily affect the overlying articular cartilage. Therefore, the primary goal of surgical treatment is to promote healing of the underlying subchondral bony sequestrum. Secondary goals include maintenance of joint congruity, rigid fixation of unstable fragments, and repair of osteochondral defects.

FIGURE 3

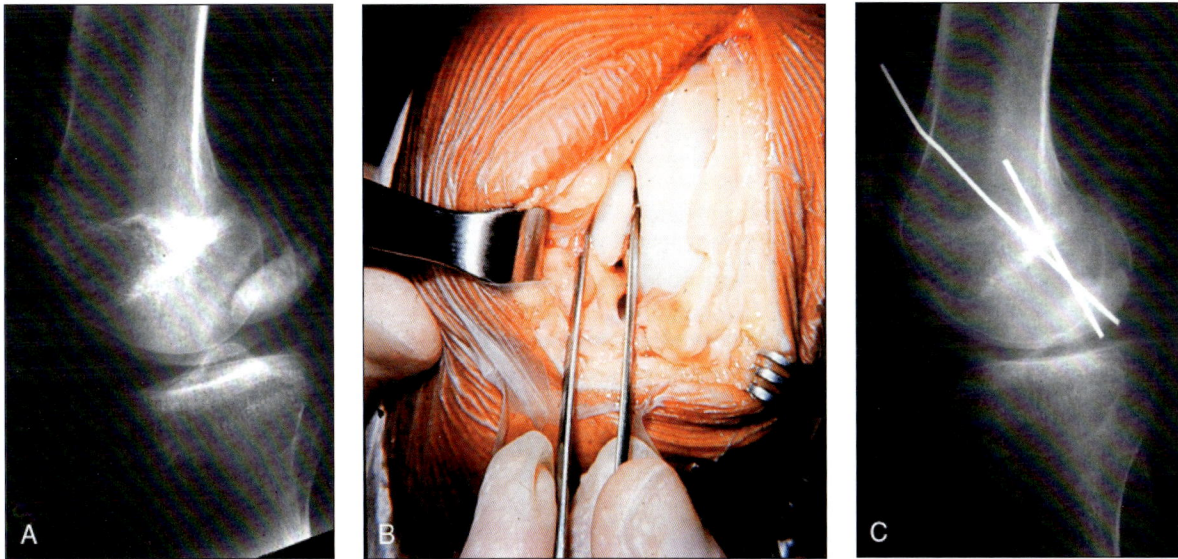

Images of an unstable osteochondritis dissecans lesion in a patient approaching skeletal maturity treated using arthrotomy, bone grafting, and K-wire fixation. **A,** Preoperative lateral radiograph. **B,** Intraoperative photograph. **C,** Lateral radiograph obtained 3 months postoperatively. (Adapted with permission from Kocher MS, Tucker R, Ganley TJ, Flynn JM: Management of osteochondritis dissecans of the knee: Current concepts review. *Am J Sports Med* 2006;34[7]:1181-1191.)

Although success with arthroscopic drilling of stable juvenile forms of OCD has been well documented in the literature,[7,16-19] this technique has had less success in the adult population. Stable intact lesions in the adult are best treated with drilling and fixation of the area affected by OCD. In cases with unstable lesions, the removal of fibrous tissue between the fragments is required. If significant portions of nonviable bone must be resected, either from the base of the defect or the fragment, autologous bone grafting should be performed before fragment reduction and fixation (**Figure 3**). Fixation can be achieved using a variety of methods, including tibial metaphyseal bone strips, bioabsorbable screws, Herbert screws, wires, and tacks.[20-23] A variety of techniques have been developed and researched for the treatment of large unsalvageable fragments including abrasionplasty, microfracture, autologous chondrocyte implantation, and osteochondral autograft and allograft transplantation.[24-27]

Expert Opinion

According to this chapter's authors, preferred treatment of OCD includes a thorough history and detailed physical examination. Diagnostic imaging should include plain radiography (AP, lateral, notch, and skyline views) followed by MRI. Stable lesions in skeletally immature patients can be treated with a three-phase nonsurgical protocol including 4 to 6 weeks of knee immobilization and crutch-protected partial weight bearing. Weeks 4 through 6 include weight bearing as tolerated without immobilization, followed by a 4- to 6-week period of rehabilitation that emphasizes knee range of motion and low-impact quadriceps and hamstring strengthening. Stable lesions for which nonsurgical management has failed and unstable lesions should be treated arthroscopically using transarticular drilling and internal fixation when indicated (articular cartilage breach). Loose and/ or fragmented defects may ultimately require arthrotomy for open fixation, bone grafting or microfracture, and possibly future chondral resurfacing procedures. Anderson and Pagnani[28] clearly demonstrated that simple excision of childhood OCD lesions ultimately results in extremely poor long-term outcomes clinically, functionally, and radiographically.

ACL INJURY

Intrasubstance ACL injuries in children and adolescents were once considered rare occurrences, with tibial eminence avulsion fractures generally regarded as equivalent to pediatric ACL injuries.[29-31] However, with increased single-sport focus and year-round training at younger ages, intrasubstance ACL injuries in children and adolescents are being diagnosed with increased frequency. As in the adult, a knee devoid of ligamentous stability predisposes the patient to meniscal and chondral injuries and early degenerative changes.

ACL injury has been reported in 10% to 65% of pediatric knees with acute traumatic hemarthrosis in series ranging from 35 to 138 patients.[12,32-36] Controversy exists regarding the management of ACL injuries in skeletally immature individuals. Although nonsurgical management of partial tears may be successful in some patients, nonsurgical management of complete tears in individuals with open physes generally has a poor prognosis, with recurrent instability leading to eventual meniscal and chondral pathology and potential early degenerative changes.[37-43] Graf et al,[38] Mizuta et al,[42] and Janarv et al[39] have reported instability symptoms, subsequent meniscal tears, decreased activity levels, and the need for ACL reconstruction in most skeletally immature patients treated nonsurgically in series of 8, 23, and 18 patients, respectively. Similarly, when comparing the results of surgical versus nonsurgical management of complete ACL injuries in adolescents, McCarroll et al[40] and Pressman et al[43] found that those injuries managed with ACL reconstruction had less instability, higher activity and return-to-sport levels, and lower rates of subsequent reinjury and meniscal tears. However, to date, no definitive evidence has been found to support the concept that ACL reconstruction forestalls the progression of osteoarthritis after an initial ACL injury.

Conventional surgical reconstruction techniques risk potential iatrogenic growth disturbance resulting from physeal violation. Cases of growth disturbance have been reported in animal models[44-46] but rarely in clinical series.[47-49] Lipscomb and Anderson[47] reported one case of 20 mm of shortening in a series of 24 skeletally immature patients who underwent reconstruction using transphyseal semitendinosus and gracilis grafts. This complication was associated with stable graft fixation across the physis.

In a survey of the Herodicus Society and the ACL Study Group, Kocher et al[50] noted 15 cases of growth disturbance ranging from distal femoral valgus deformity to tibial recurvatum to limb-length discrepancy (2 cases). Associated factors included fixation hardware across the physis, bone plugs across the physis, large (12-mm) tunnels, and suturing near the tibial tubercle apophysis.

Surgical techniques used to treat ACL insufficiency in skeletally immature patients include primary repair, extra-articular tenodesis, transphyseal reconstruction, partial transphyseal reconstruction, and physeal-sparing reconstruction. Primary repair and extra-articular tenodesis alone have shown poor results in children and adolescents, similar to results in adults.[38,40,50,51] Transphyseal reconstructions with tunnels that violate both the distal femoral and proximal tibial physes have been performed using a variety of grafts with good to excellent short-term outcomes.[37,40,52-55] Partial transphyseal reconstructions include all epiphyseal techniques,[56-58] whereas a variety of physeal-sparing reconstructions have been described in the literature.[34,59-63] It is important to remember that not all skeletally immature patients are the same; therefore, a single approach cannot be used to surgically reconstruct every pediatric ACL.

Adult Sequelae

Adult ACL insufficiency presents in a fashion similar to that in the skeletally immature individual with a ruptured ACL. Both contact and noncontact twisting injuries can precipitate an audible pop with subsequent knee effusions. Primary symptoms include instability, giving way, and difficulty bearing weight.

Physical examination must begin with an inspection of the patient's gait. A quadriceps avoidance gait is often noted in patients with acute or chronic ACL injuries. Subsequent evaluation of the knee depends on a relaxed and cooperative patient. Range of motion must be assessed. Ligamentous laxity must be evaluated by using the Lachman, pivot-shift, and anterior drawer tests. The remaining knee ligaments must be evaluated and the menisci thoroughly examined (for example, using varus/valgus laxity, joint line tenderness, and the Steinmann and McMurray tests). Comparison with the contralateral knee often can be helpful in equivocal examinations.

Diagnostic imaging should include plain radiography (AP and lateral views are sufficient) and MRI. These imaging studies are important to rule out other abnormalities and associated injuries. A vertically oriented Segond fracture, often associated with an ACL injury, results from excessive tension on the lateral capsular ligaments of the knee. MRI has high sensitivity and specificity for intra-articular knee pathologies, especially ACL injuries. These injuries can be seen in greatest detail on both T1- and T2-weighted sagittal images. In acute injuries, the traditional bone contusion pattern of ACL injuries can be seen (the central third of the lateral femoral condyle, the posterior third of the lateral tibial plateau). Other internal derangements (such as meniscal injuries or chondral defects) can be detected on MRI and subsequently treated during arthroscopic intervention.

Interventions for the Adult Patient

Nonsurgical treatment of complete ACL ruptures should be reserved for only a select group of patients, including, but not limited to, elderly patients, nonathletic individuals willing to avoid high-risk activities, and those with preexisting advanced knee arthritis or joint sepsis. Two randomized controlled trials in the late 1980s and early 1990s in Sweden compared nonsurgical treatment of ACL tears with repair/reconstruction. All studies found higher validated outcome scores after reconstruction compared with nonsurgical treatment, but concluded that in less active individuals willing to forego high-risk activities, nonsurgical treatment was feasible.[64,65] Nonsurgical therapy includes bracing, rehabilitation (emphasizing quadriceps and hamstring strengthening as well as neuromuscular and proprioceptive training), and activity modification.

The goal of surgical management is to restore the functional stability of the knee, with near-anatomic reconstruction of the ACL to forestall the progression of meniscal tears, chondral injuries, and eventually, early degenerative changes.[66-68] Bottoni et al[69] clearly demonstrated a marked benefit of waiting 2 to 4 weeks between

ACL rupture and reconstruction. In comparing early versus delayed reconstruction, the authors noted that surgery in the acute setting (<3 weeks) increases the risk of arthrofibrosis and additional procedures. Surgical considerations include age, activity level, pain tolerance, rehabilitation potential, cosmesis, and the surgeon's graft and technical preference. Graft options include allograft and autograft, and may be harvested from the patellar tendon and hamstrings. No level I randomized controlled trials exist comparing allograft with autograft reconstruction, although a variety of cohort studies indicate no significant difference in final outcomes or morbidity.[70] Borchers et al[71] recently demonstrated that higher activity levels after reconstruction and the use of allograft are risk factors for ACL graft failure. A variety of graft fixation options are available; each has advantages and disadvantages. More aggressive return-to-play and rehabilitation programs are now available, emphasizing graft fixation complexes with superior mechanical and biologic fixation.[72,73] Traditional 3- and 6-month postoperative rehabilitation programs for return to in-line jogging and pivoting sports, respectively, are continually being revised and advanced.

Expert Opinion

According to this chapter's authors, preferred treatment of ACL reconstruction in skeletally immature patients includes a thorough history and a detailed physical examination, along with evaluation of ligamentous stability and other associated knee pathology. Preoperative planning should include a determination of both skeletal and physiologic age (**Table 1**). Radiographs of the hand and wrist are obtained to determine skeletal age. Radiographs of the knee also are routinely obtained. MRI of the knee is frequently used to determine the presence of associated injuries such as meniscal tears and chondral injuries. In skeletally immature patients, as in adult patients, acute ACL reconstructions are not performed within the first 3 weeks after injury to minimize the risk of arthrofibrosis. Preoperative rehabilitation is used to regain range of motion, minimize swelling, and maximize strength.

The type of reconstruction procedure is dictated by the patient's physiologic and skeletal age (**Figure 4**). In prepubescent skeletally immature individuals, a physeal-sparing procedure is combined with intra-articular and

TABLE 1 Tanner Classification of Secondary Sexual Characteristics

Tanner Stage	Male	Female
Stage 1 (prepubertal)		
Growth	5–6 cm/y	5–6 cm/y
Development	Testes <4 mL or <2.5 cm, no pubic hair	No breast development, no pubic hair
Stage 2		
Growth	5–6 cm/y	7–8 cm/y
Development	Testes 4 mL or 2.5–3.2 cm, minimal pubic hair at base of penis	Breast buds, minimal pubic hair on labia
Stage 3		
Growth	7–8 cm/y	8 cm/y
Development	Testes 12 mL or 3.6 cm, pubic hair over pubis, voice changes, muscle mass increases	Elevation of breast, areolae enlarge; pubic hair on mons pubis, axillary hair, acne
Stage 4		
Growth	10 cm/y	7 cm/y
Development	Testes 4.1–4.5 cm, pubic hair as adult, axillary hair, acne	Areolae enlarge, pubic hair as adult
Stage 5		
Growth	No growth	No growth
Development	Testes as adult, pubic hair as adult, facial hair as adult, mature physique	Adult breast contour, pubic hair as adult
Other	Peak height velocity: 13.5 years	Adrenarche: 6–8 years, menarche: 12.7 years, peak height velocity: 11.5 years

Data adapted from Guzzanti V, Falciglia F, Stanitski CL: Preoperative evaluation and anterior cruciate ligament reconstruction technique for skeletally immature patients in Tanner stages 2 and 3. *Am J Sports Med* 2003;31(6):941-948.

extra-articular reconstruction using an iliotibial band graft[74] (**Figure 5**). In adolescent patients with growth remaining (open physes), a transphyseal reconstruction with hamstrings tendon graft and metaphyseal fixation is used.[75] In older adolescents with closed physes, an adult ACL reconstruction with interference screw fixation is performed as it would be in an adult using either a central third bone–patellar tendon–bone graft or a hamstrings tendon graft. Postoperative rehabilitation is then specific to the type of reconstruction performed.

MENISCAL TEARS

The reported incidence of meniscal tears in skeletally immature patients has increased in recent years, likely because of increased sports participation and more accurate diagnostic modalities including MRI.[76] Traumatic meniscal injuries in children younger than 10 years typically occur in the setting of discoid meniscus. In older children and adolescents, most non–discoid meniscus tears often are the result of twisting injuries sustained during sports activity.

Stanitski et al[35] noted meniscal tears in 47% of preadolescents (age range, 7 to 12 years) and in 45% of adolescents (age range, 13 to 18 years) with acute traumatic hemarthrosis of the knee. In both groups, the medial meniscus was more likely to be torn (70% for preadolescents, 88% for adolescents). In the adolescent group, a concurrent ACL tear occurred in 36% of cases. Of all meniscal tears sustained by adolescent patients, 50% involve the periphery of the meniscus and are thus more

FIGURE 4

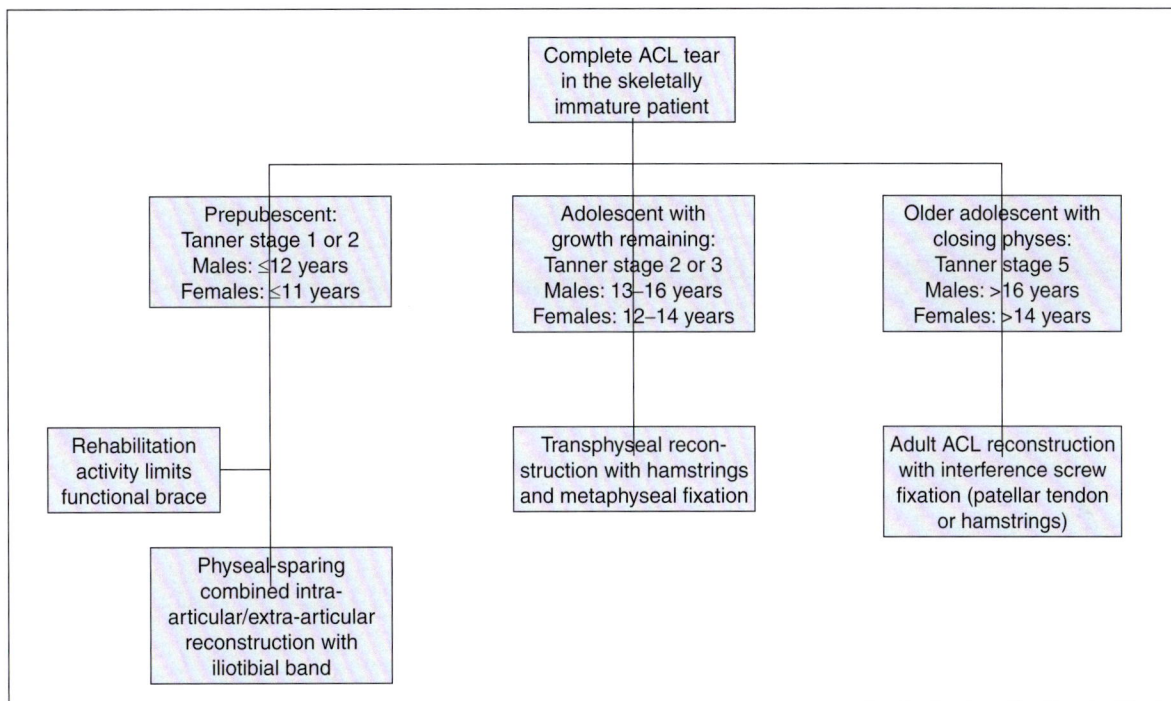

Algorithm for management of complete anterior cruciate ligament (ACL) injuries in skeletally immature patients. (Adapted with permission from: Kocher MS: Reconstruction of the anterior cruciate ligament in the skeletally immature patient. *Oper Tech Orthop* 2005;15:298-307.)

amenable to repair, as opposed to resection.

The developing meniscus in the skeletally immature individual has a unique vascularity, histologic structure, and biomechanical composition contributing to its increased healing potential.[77] Moreover, most meniscal tears in children occur in the periphery (red-red zone) as longitudinal tears; in adults, a preponderance of degenerative cleavage tears occur at the inner meniscal rim. As a result, attention should be directed toward repair of all meniscal injuries in the preadolescent and adolescent age groups when possible. Treatment options include resection, repair, allograft transplantation, and, in the case of discoid meniscus, saucerization.

Cadaver studies have demonstrated that with partial meniscectomy of the medial meniscus, contact pressures increase by 65% in the medial compartment, and with total meniscectomy, stresses increase by 235%.[78,79] Manzione et al[80] clearly demonstrated deleterious out-

comes after complete or partial meniscectomy in children at long-term follow-up. At 5-year follow-up, 75% of patients were symptomatic, 80% had radiographic evidence of early degenerative changes, and 60% were dissatisfied with their results. In a more recent review, Lohmander et al[81] noted that 50% of patients who underwent total meniscectomy had radiographic changes, symptoms, and functional loss consistent with osteoarthritis at 10- to 20-year follow-up. As a result, meniscal repair is favored over meniscectomy in children with symptomatic meniscal tears to prevent any progression toward the early onset of arthritis.

Adult Sequelae

Meniscal pathology can present differently in adults than in children. Although a child with discoid meniscus might report snapping, inability to fully extend the knee, and lateral knee pain, an adult typically presents

FIGURE 5

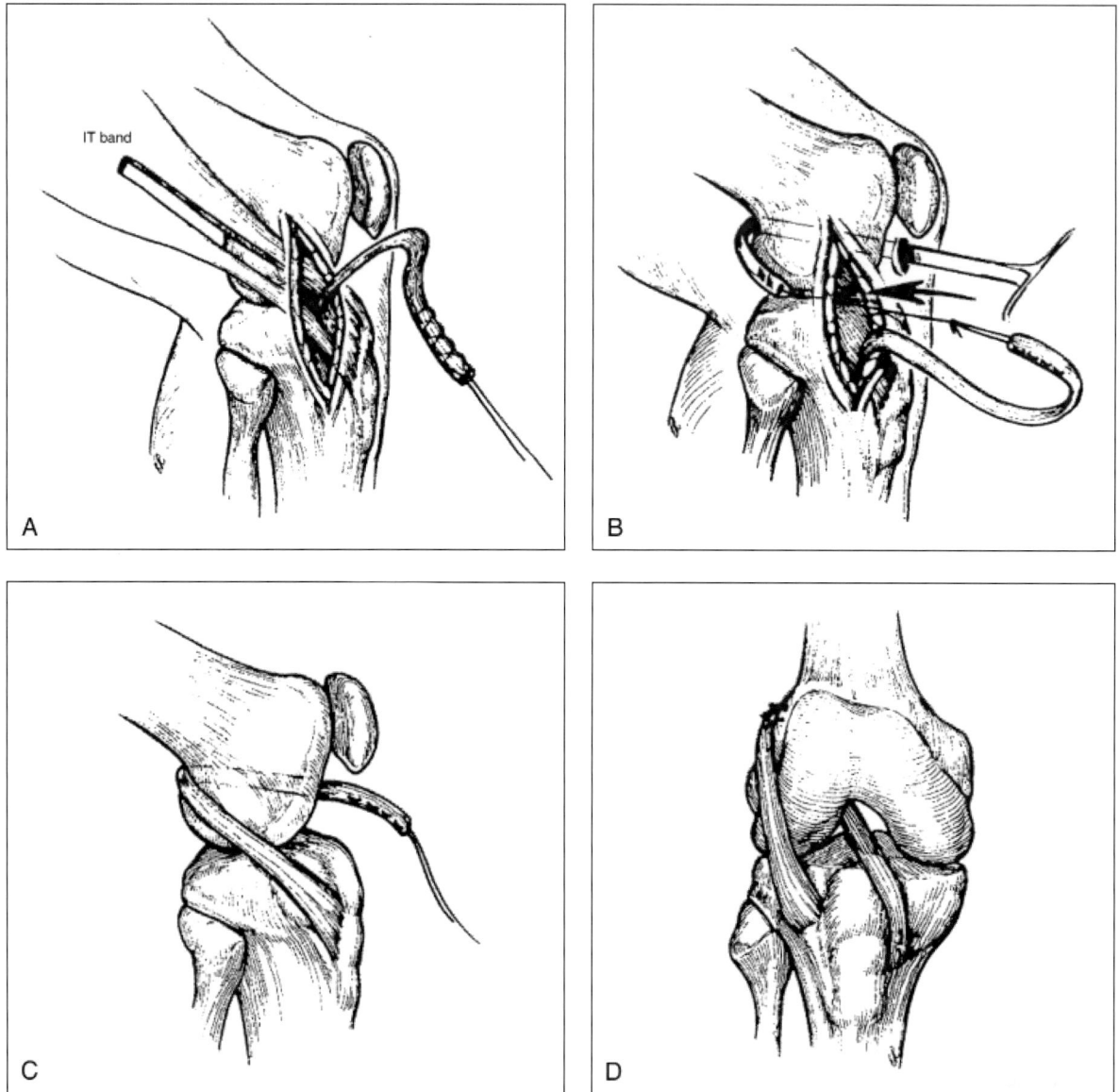

Illustrations show physeal-sparing intra-articular and extra-articular combined reconstruction using autologous iliotibial band for prepubescent patients. **A,** The iliotibial band graft is harvested free proximally and left attached to the Gerdy tubercle distally. **B,** The graft is brought through the knee in the over-the-top position posteriorly (arrow). **C,** The graft is brought through the knee and under the intermeniscal ligament anteriorly. **D,** Resultant intra-articular and extra-articular reconstruction. (Adapted with permission from Kocher MS: Reconstruction of the anterior cruciate ligament in the skeletally immature patient. *Oper Tech Orthop* 2005;15:298-307.)

with pain, stiffness, locking, and swelling: both presentations warrant further investigation. Physical examination of the adult knee must include evaluation for effusion, assessment for range of motion, joint line palpation for tenderness, and provocative maneuvers to elicit signs of meniscal pain (the McMurray, Steinmann, and Apley tests). Weinstabl et al[82] found that joint line tenderness was the best clinical sign of a meniscal tear, with 74% sensitivity and a 50% positive predictive value.

Diagnostic workup begins with radiography of the knee (typically four views are obtained: AP, lateral, notch, and skyline). Notch views are necessary to rule out other bony pathologies such as OCD and early degenerative changes as the source of knee pain. Patellar subluxation also must be considered with lateral joint pain. MRI is advantageous because of its noninvasive nature, its ability to image the knee in multiple planes, the absence of ionizing radiation, and its capacity for the evaluation of other structures within the knee joint. The limitations of MRI include a relatively high cost to health care and the patient as well as the potential for misinterpreting nonpathologic entities. In 1997, Muellner et al[83] noted 80% to 90% accuracy in using MRI for the detection of meniscal tears. However, in the child, the posterior horn of the medial meniscus often demonstrates increased vascularity, which can be misinterpreted as a tear. With the advent of higher-powered magnets such as the 3-Tesla (T3), multiple radiology-based articles have purported this number to now approach greater than 95% accuracy. Even with such powerful imaging tools, integrating the history, physical examination, and diagnostic workup is still critical in making treatment recommendations.

Interventions for the Adult Patient

Nonsurgical treatment of meniscal tears in the adult patient should be reserved for largely asymptomatic lesions that have minimal effect on activities of daily living. Once mechanical symptoms and pain or effusion become persistent, surgical intervention is warranted. The spectrum of surgical treatment includes partial meniscectomy, meniscal repair, and meniscal allograft transplantation.

Many adult meniscal lesions are degenerative tears of the inner third of the meniscus. In the red-white and white-white zones, meniscal repair becomes exceed-

ingly difficult and partial menisectomy is the preferred treatment. Metcalf et al[84] proposed general guidelines for arthroscopic resection of meniscal lesions that include the following: (1) All mobile fragments that can be pulled past the inner margin of the meniscus into the center of the joint should be removed. (2) The remaining meniscal rim should be smoothed to remove any sudden changes in contour that might lead to further tearing. (3) A perfectly smooth rim is not necessary. Repeat arthroscopy has shown rim remodeling and smoothing at 6 to 9 months. (4) The probe should be used repeatedly to gain information about the mobility and texture of the remaining rim. (5) The meniscocapsular junction and the peripheral meniscal rim should be protected. This maintains meniscal stability and is vital in preserving the load transmission properties of the meniscus. (6) To optimize efficiency, both manual and motorized resection instruments should be used. (7) In uncertain situations, more of the meniscal rim should be left intact to avoid segmental resection, which essentially results in subtotal menisectomy, particularly in lateral meniscal tears.

Meniscal repair should be used for any peripheral tear in the red-red zone or amenable tear patterns in the red-white zone, including longitudinal tears and viable bucket-handle lesions. Repair techniques include inside-out sutures, outside-in sutures, and a variety of all-inside fixation techniques and methods. For all techniques, the first step is to prepare the meniscus with meticulous débridement of the loose edges of the tear and rasping the perimeniscal synovium.[85] This achieves reduction of the tear, followed by adequate stabilization using one of many fixation methods. Vertical mattress inside-out sutures are considered the gold standard for repair. Posteromedial and posterolateral incisions are used with this technique to prevent injury to the saphenous and sural nerves, respectively. Numerous all-inside devices on the market include bioabsorbable screws, darts, arrows, and anchors. Biomechanical testing has demonstrated superior fixation with meniscal repair systems. Suture-based flexible and low-profile devices that allow compression across the tear site and minimize injury to the adjacent chondral surfaces are ideal.

Meniscal allograft transplantation is a relatively new reconstruction procedure and can be medial or lateral. Medial allografts are typically connected using anterior and posterior bone plugs, whereas lateral allografts are inserted using an accompanying bone slot. Although the indications for menisal allograft transplantation continue to increase, current ideal indications include near-total or total menisectomy and joint line pain, early chondral changes, normal anatomic alignment, and a ligamentously stable knee.[86] Corrective osteotomy and/or ligamentous reconstruction can be performed concurrently with meniscal allograft transplantation in certain cases. Limited long-term data exist to definitively support using meniscal allograft transplantation; however, in patients with severe injury and irreparable meniscal tissue, meniscal allograft transplantation may be the patient's only viable option.

Expert Opinion

According to this chapter's authors, preferred treatment of meniscal injuries in skeletally immature patients includes a thorough history and physical examination, along with evaluation for symptoms of discoid meniscus. Subsequent imaging should include radiography (AP, lateral, notch, and skyline views) followed by MRI. Associated injuries including chondral defects and loose bodies must be ruled out.

For a meniscal tear in the child's knee, every effort must be made to repair the meniscus before performing a partial menisectomy. Tears of the posterior horn are traditionally treated using an inside-out repair, whereas anterior horn lesions can be addressed using either an open or an outside-in technique (for example, the Mulberry knot). All-inside fixation methods have become more reliable and biomechanically sturdy. For a near-total menisectomy with early degenerative changes and normal alignment and ligamentous stability, meniscal allograft transplantation can be considered, even in skeletally immature individuals. Postoperative rehabilitation encompasses partial weight bearing in a hinged range-of-motion brace. Range of motion is initially restricted to 0° to 40° and gradually increased to 0° to 90° by 6 weeks postoperatively. Return to play is allowed at 3 to 4 months postoperatively.[77]

CONCLUSION

Osteochondritis dissecans, ACL injury, and meniscal tears are increasingly common complications for the young athlete. Nonsurgical treatment can often lead to debilitating consequences and early degenerative changes as an adult. Prompt diagnosis, safe and effective treatment, and gradual return to play are all critical factors in forestalling the potential progression to early degenerative changes.

REFERENCES

1. Kocher MS, Tucker R, Ganley TJ, Flynn JM: Management of osteochondritis dissecans of the knee: Current concepts review. *Am J Sports Med* 2006;34(7):1181-1191.

2. Lindén B: The incidence of osteochondritis dissecans in the condyles of the femur. *Acta Orthop Scand* 1976;47(6):664-667.

3. Crawford DC, Safran MR: Osteochondritis dissecans of the knee. *J Am Acad Orthop Surg* 2006;14(2):90-100.

4. Hefti F, Beguiristain J, Krauspe R, et al: Osteochondritis dissecans: A multicenter study of the European Pediatric Orthopedic Society. *J Pediatr Orthop B* 1999;8(4):231-245.

5. Cahill BR: Osteochondritis dissecans of the knee: Treatment of juvenile and adult forms. *J Am Acad Orthop Surg* 1995;3(4):237-247.

6. Wall EJ, Vourazeris J, Myer GD, et al: The healing potential of stable juvenile osteochondritis dissecans knee lesions. *J Bone Joint Surg Am* 2008;90(12):2655-2664.

7. Kocher MS, Micheli LJ, Yaniv M, Zurakowski D, Ames A, Adrignolo AA: Functional and radiographic outcome of juvenile osteochondritis dissecans of the knee treated with transarticular arthroscopic drilling. *Am J Sports Med* 2001;29(5):562-566.

8. Kocher MS, Czarnecki JJ, Andersen JS, Micheli LJ: Internal fixation of juvenile osteochondritis dissecans lesions of the knee. *Am J Sports Med* 2007;35(5):712-718.

9. Conrad JM, Stanitski CL: Osteochondritis dissecans: Wilson's sign revisited. *Am J Sports Med* 2003;31(5):777-778.

10. Cahill BR, Berg BC: 99m-Technetium phosphate compound joint scintigraphy in the management of juvenile osteochondritis dissecans of the femoral condyles. *Am J Sports Med* 1983;11(5):329-335.

11. Cahill BR, Phillips MR, Navarro R: The results of conservative management of juvenile osteochondritis dissecans using joint scintigraphy: A prospective study. *Am J Sports Med* 1989;17(5):601-606.

12. Kocher MS, DiCanzio J, Zurakowski D, Micheli LJ: Diagnostic performance of clinical examination and selective magnetic resonance imaging in the evaluation

of intraarticular knee disorders in children and adolescents. *Am J Sports Med* 2001;29(3):292-296.

13. Pill SG, Ganley TJ, Milam RA, Lou JE, Meyer JS, Flynn JM: Role of magnetic resonance imaging and clinical criteria in predicting successful nonoperative treatment of osteochondritis dissecans in children. *J Pediatr Orthop* 2003;23(1):102-108.

14. Garrett JC: Osteochondritis dissecans. *Clin Sports Med* 1991;10(3):569-593.

15. Smillie IS: Treatment of osteochondritis dissecans. *J Bone Joint Surg Br* 1957;39-B(2):248-260.

16. Aglietti P, Buzzi R, Bassi PB, Fioriti M: Arthroscopic drilling in juvenile osteochondritis dissecans of the medial femoral condyle. *Arthroscopy* 1994;10(3):286-291.

17. Bradley J, Dandy DJ: Results of drilling osteochondritis dissecans before skeletal maturity. *J Bone Joint Surg Br* 1989;71(4):642-644.

18. Anderson AF, Richards DB, Pagnani MJ, Hovis WD: Antegrade drilling for osteochondritis dissecans of the knee. *Arthroscopy* 1997;13(3):319-324.

19. Ganley TJ, Amro RR, Gregg JR: Antegrade drilling for osteochondritis dissecans of the knee. P*ediatric Orthopaedic Society of North America 2002 Annual Meeting*. Salt Lake City, UT, 2002.

20. Cugat R, Garcia M, Cusco X, et al: Osteochondritis dissecans: A historical review and its treatment with cannulated screws. *Arthroscopy* 1993;9(6):675-684.

21. Johnson LL, Uitvlugt G, Austin MD, Detrisac DA, Johnson C: Osteochondritis dissecans of the knee: Arthroscopic compression screw fixation. *Arthroscopy* 1990;6(3):179-189.

22. Navarro R, Cohen M, Filho MC, da Silva RT: The arthroscopic treatment of osteochondritis dissecans of the knee with autologous bone sticks. *Arthroscopy* 2002;18(8):840-844.

23. Rey Zuniga JJ, Sagastibelza J, Lopez Blasco JJ, Martinez Grande M: Arthroscopic use of the Herbert screw in osteochondritis dissecans of the knee. *Arthroscopy* 1993;9(6):668-670.

24. Bentley G, Biant LC, Carrington RW, et al: A prospective, randomised comparison of autologous chondrocyte implantation versus mosaicplasty for osteochondral defects in the knee. *J Bone Joint Surg Br* 2003;85(2):223-230.

25. Berlet GC, Mascia A, Miniaci A: Treatment of unstable osteochondritis dissecans lesions of the knee using autogenous osteochondral grafts (mosaicplasty). *Arthroscopy* 1999;15(3):312-316.

26. Madsen BL, Noer HH, Carstensen JP, Nørmark F: Long-term results of periosteal transplantation in osteochondritis dissecans of the knee. *Orthopedics* 2000;23(3):223-226.

27. Yoshizumi Y, Sugita T, Kawamata T, Ohnuma M, Maeda S: Cylindrical osteochondral graft for osteochondritis dissecans of the knee: A report of three cases. *Am J Sports Med* 2002;30(3):441-445.

28. Anderson AF, Pagnani MJ: Osteochondritis dissecans of the femoral condyles: Long-term results of excision of the fragment. *Am J Sports Med* 1997;25(6):830-834.

29. Kocher MS, Micheli LJ, Gerbino P, Hresko MT: Tibial eminence fractures in children: Prevalence of meniscal entrapment. *Am J Sports Med* 2003;31(3):404-407.

30. Kocher MS, Foreman ES, Micheli LJ: Laxity and functional outcome after arthroscopic reduction and internal fixation of displaced tibial spine fractures in children. *Arthroscopy* 2003;19(10):1085-1090.

31. Kocher MS, Mandiga R, Klingele K, Bley L, Micheli LJ: Anterior cruciate ligament injury versus tibial spine fracture in the skeletally immature knee: A comparison of skeletal maturation and notch width index. *J Pediatr Orthop* 2004;24(2):185-188.

32. Eiskjaer S, Larsen ST, Schmidt MB: The significance of hemarthrosis of the knee in children. *Arch Orthop Trauma Surg* 1988;107(2):96-98.

33. Kloeppel-Wirth S, Koltai JL, Dittmer H: Significance of arthroscopy in children with knee joint injuries. *Eur J Pediatr Surg* 1992;2(3):169-172.

34. Vähäsarja V, Kinnuen P, Serlo W: Arthroscopy of the acute traumatic knee in children: Prospective study of 138 cases. *Acta Orthop Scand* 1993;64(5):580-582.

35. Stanitski CL, Harvell JC, Fu F: Observations on acute knee hemarthrosis in children and adolescents. *J Pediatr Orthop* 1993;13(4):506-510.

36. Luhmann SJ: Acute traumatic knee effusions in children and adolescents. *J Pediatr Orthop* 2003;23(2):199-202.

37. Aichroth PM, Patel DV, Zorrilla P: The natural history and treatment of rupture of the anterior cruciate ligament in children and adolescents: A prospective review. *J Bone Joint Surg Br* 2002;84(1):38-41.

38. Graf BK, Lange RH, Fujisaki CK, Landry GL, Saluja RK: Anterior cruciate ligament tears in skeletally immature patients: Meniscal pathology at presentation and

after attempted conservative treatment. *Arthroscopy* 1992;8(2):229-233.

39. Janarv PM, Nyström A, Werner S, Hirsch G: Anterior cruciate ligament injuries in skeletally immature patients. *J Pediatr Orthop* 1996;16(5):673-677.

40. McCarroll JR, Rettig AC, Shelbourne KD: Anterior cruciate ligament injuries in the young athlete with open physes. *Am J Sports Med* 1988;16(1):44-47.

41. Millett PJ, Willis AA, Warren RF: Associated injuries in pediatric and adolescent anterior cruciate ligament tears: Does a delay in treatment increase the risk of meniscal tear? *Arthroscopy* 2002;18(9):955-959.

42. Mizuta H, Kubota K, Shiraishi M, Otsuka Y, Nagamoto N, Takagi K: The conservative treatment of complete tears of the anterior cruciate ligament in skeletally immature patients. *J Bone Joint Surg Br* 1995;77(6):890-894.

43. Pressman AE, Letts RM, Jarvis JG: Anterior cruciate ligament tears in children: An analysis of operative versus nonoperative treatment. *J Pediatr Orthop* 1997;17(4):505-511.

44. Guzzanti V, Falciglia F, Gigante A, Fabbriciani C: The effect of intra-articular ACL reconstruction on the growth plates of rabbits. *J Bone Joint Surg Br* 1994;76(6):960-963.

45. Houle JB, Letts M, Yang J: Effects of a tensioned tendon graft in a bone tunnel across the rabbit physis. *Clin Orthop Relat Res* 2001(391):275-281.

46. Edwards TB, Greene CC, Baratta RV, Zieske A, Willis RB: The effect of placing a tensioned graft across open growth plates: A gross and histologic analysis. *J Bone Joint Surg Am* 2001;83-A(5):725-734.

47. Lipscomb AB, Anderson AF: Tears of the anterior cruciate ligament in adolescents. *J Bone Joint Surg Am* 1986;68(1):19-28.

48. Koman JD, Sanders JO: Valgus deformity after reconstruction of the anterior cruciate ligament in a skeletally immature patient: A case report. *J Bone Joint Surg Am* 1999;81(5):711-715.

49. Kocher MS, Saxon HS, Hovis WD, Hawkins RJ: Management and complications of anterior cruciate ligament injuries in skeletally immature patients: Survey of the Herodicus Society and The ACL Study Group. *J Pediatr Orthop* 2002;22(4):452-457.

50. Clanton TO, DeLee JC, Sanders B, Neidre A: Knee ligament injuries in children. *J Bone Joint Surg Am* 1979;61(8):1195-1201.

51. Engebretsen L, Svenningsen S, Benum P: Poor results of anterior cruciate ligament repair in adolescence. *Acta Orthop Scand* 1988;59(6):684-686.

52. Angel KR, Hall DJ: Anterior cruciate ligament injury in children and adolescents. *Arthroscopy* 1989;5(3):197-200.

53. Aronowitz ER, Ganley TJ, Goode JR, Gregg JR, Meyer JS: Anterior cruciate ligament reconstruction in adolescents with open physes. *Am J Sports Med* 2000;28(2):168-175.

54. Fuchs R, Wheatley W, Uribe JW, Hechtman KS, Zvijac JE, Schurhoff MR: Intra-articular anterior cruciate ligament reconstruction using patellar tendon allograft in the skeletally immature patient. *Arthroscopy* 2002;18(8):824-828.

55. Matava MJ, Siegel MG: Arthroscopic reconstruction of the ACL with semitendinosus-gracilis autograft in skeletally immature adolescent patients. *Am J Knee Surg* 1997;10(2):60-69.

56. Andrews M, Noyes FR, Barber-Westin SD: Anterior cruciate ligament allograft reconstruction in the skeletally immature athlete. *Am J Sports Med* 1994;22(1):48-54.

57. Bisson LJ, Wickiewicz T, Levinson M, Warren R: ACL reconstruction in children with open physes. *Orthopedics* 1998;21(6):659-663.

58. Guzzanti V, Falciglia F, Stanitski CL: Preoperative evaluation and anterior cruciate ligament reconstruction technique for skeletally immature patients in Tanner stages 2 and 3. *Am J Sports Med* 2003;31(6):941-948.

59. Brief LP: Anterior cruciate ligament reconstruction without drill holes. *Arthroscopy* 1991;7(4):350-357.

60. DeLee JC, Curtis R: Anterior cruciate ligament insufficiency in children. *Clin Orthop Relat Res* 1983(172):112-118.

61. Kim SH, Ha KI, Ahn JH, Chang DK: Anterior cruciate ligament reconstruction in the young patient without violation of the epiphyseal plate. *Arthroscopy* 1999;15(7):792-795.

62. Parker AW, Drez D Jr, Cooper JL: Anterior cruciate ligament injuries in patients with open physes. *Am J Sports Med* 1994;22(1):44-47.

63. Anderson AF: Transepiphyseal replacement of the anterior cruciate ligament in skeletally immature patients: A preliminary report. *J Bone Joint Surg Am* 2003;85A(7):1255-1263.

64. Andersson C, Odensten M, Gillquist J: Knee function after surgical or nonsurgical treatment of acute rupture

of the anterior cruciate ligament: A randomized study with a long-term follow-up period. *Clin Orthop Relat Res* 1991(264):255-263.

65. Andersson C, Odensten M, Good L, Gillquist J: Surgical or non-surgical treatment of acute rupture of the anterior cruciate ligament: A randomized study with long-term follow-up. *J Bone Joint Surg Am* 1989;71(7):965-974.

66. Levy AS, Meier SW: Approach to cartilage injury in the anterior cruciate ligament-deficient knee. *Orthop Clin North Am* 2003;34(1):149-167.

67. Beynnon BD, Johnson RJ, Abate JA, Fleming BC, Nichols CE: Treatment of anterior cruciate ligament injuries, part 2. *Am J Sports Med* 2005;33(11):1751-1767.

68. Beynnon BD, Johnson RJ, Abate JA, Fleming BC, Nichols CE: Treatment of anterior cruciate ligament injuries, part I. *Am J Sports Med* 2005;33(10):1579-1602.

69. Bottoni CR, Liddell TR, Trainor TJ, Freccero DM, Lindell KK: Postoperative range of motion following anterior cruciate ligament reconstruction using autograft hamstrings: A prospective, randomized clinical trial of early versus delayed reconstructions. *Am J Sports Med* 2008;36(4):656-662.

70. Baer GS, Harner CD: Clinical outcomes of allograft versus autograft in anterior cruciate ligament reconstruction. *Clin Sports Med* 2007;26(4):661-681.

71. Borchers JR, Pedroza A, Kaeding C: Activity level and graft type as risk factors for anterior cruciate ligament graft failure: A case-control study. *Am J Sports Med* 2009;37(12):2362-2367.

72. Milano G, Mulas PD, Ziranu F, Piras S, Manunta A, Fabbriciani C: Comparison between different femoral fixation devices for ACL reconstruction with doubled hamstring tendon graft: A biomechanical analysis. *Arthroscopy* 2006;22(6):660-668.

73. Ahmad CS, Gardner TR, Groh M, Arnouk J, Levine WN: Mechanical properties of soft tissue femoral fixation devices for anterior cruciate ligament reconstruction. *Am J Sports Med* 2004;32(3):635-640.

74. Kocher MS, Garg S, Micheli LJ: Physeal sparing reconstruction of the anterior cruciate ligament in skeletally immature prepubescent children and adolescents. *J Bone Joint Surg Am* 2005;87(11):2371-2379.

75. Kocher MS, Smith JT, Zoric BJ, Lee B, Micheli LJ: Transphyseal anterior cruciate ligament reconstruction in skeletally immature pubescent adolescents. *J Bone Joint Surg Am* 2007;89(12):2632-2639.

76. Brown TD, Davis JT: Meniscal injury in the skeletally immature patient, in Micheli LJ, Kocher MS, eds: *The Pediatric and Adolescent Knee.* Philadelphia, PA, Elsevier, 2006, pp 236-259.

77. Kramer DE, Micheli LJ: Meniscal tears and discoid meniscus in children: diagnosis and treatment. *J Am Acad Orthop Surg* 2009;17(11):698-707.

78. Fu F, Baratz ME: Meniscal injuries, in DeLee JC, Drez, D, eds: *Orthopaedic Sports Medicine: Principles and Practice.* Philadelphia, PA, WB Saunders, 1994, pp 1146-1162.

79. Baratz ME, Fu FH, Mengato R: Meniscal tears: The effect of meniscectomy and of repair on intraarticular contact areas and stress in the human knee. A preliminary report. *Am J Sports Med* 1986;14(4):270-275.

80. Manzione M, Pizzutillo PD, Peoples AB, Schweizer PA: Meniscectomy in children: A long-term follow-up study. *Am J Sports Med* 1983;11(3):111-115.

81. Lohmander LS, Englund PM, Dahl LL, Roos EM: The long-term consequence of anterior cruciate ligament and meniscus injuries: Osteoarthritis. *Am J Sports Med* 2007;35(10):1756-1769.

82. Weinstabl R, Muellner T, Vécsei V, Kainberger F, Kramer M: Economic considerations for the diagnosis and therapy of meniscal lesions: Can magnetic resonance imaging help reduce the expense? *World J Surg* 1997;21(4):363-368.

83. Muellner T, Weinstabl R, Schabus R, Vécsei V, Kainberger F: The diagnosis of meniscal tears in athletes: A comparison of clinical and magnetic resonance imaging investigations. *Am J Sports Med* 1997;25(1):7-12.

84. Metcalf RW, Burks RT, Metcalf MS, McGinty JB: Arthroscopic meniscectomy, in McGinty JB, Caspari RB, Jackson RW, Poehling, GG, eds: *Operative Arthroscopy,* ed 2. Philadelphia, PA, Lippincott-Raven, 1996, pp 263-297.

85. DeHaven KE: Meniscus repair. *Am J Sports Med* 1999;27(2):242-250.

86. Greis PE, Holmstrom MC, Bardana DD, Burks RT: Meniscal injury: II. Management. *J Am Acad Orthop Surg* 2002;10(3):177-187.

CLUBFOOT

WEN CHAO, MD

SATHEESH KUMAR RAMINENI, MD

INTRODUCTION

The term clubfoot refers to congenital talipes equinovarus, a deformity of the foot consisting of four components: forefoot adductus, midfoot cavus, hindfoot varus, and ankle equinus. Idiopathic clubfoot most commonly occurs as an isolated birth defect.[1] The prevalence of additional congenital anomalies or chromosomal abnormalities ranges from 24% to 50%.[2] The most common known etiologies of clubfoot include arthrogryposis multiplex congenita and myelomeningocele.[3] Increasing evidence shows that clubfoot severity and treatment outcomes vary by etiology. Identifying the etiology of clubfoot helps determine both the prognosis and the selection of appropriate treatment methods for the individual patient.[4]

INCIDENCE OF PEDIATRIC CONDITION

Clubfoot is one of the most common musculoskeletal birth defects. The incidence varies widely with respect to race and sex, ranging from 0.39 per 1,000 live births among the Chinese population, to 1.2 per 1,000 live births among Caucasians, to 6.8 per 1,000 live births among Polynesians.[5] Lochmiller et al[6] reported the male-to-female ratio as 2.5:1. It is becoming increasingly clear that clubfoot is multifactorial in origin. The influence of genetic factors is suggested by the various incidences among race, sex, and family history. Approximately 25% of affected individuals have a family history of idiopathic talipes equinovarus. The concordance rate for monozygotic twins is 32.5% but only 2.9% for dizygotic twins. Other etiologies of clubfoot include histologic, muscular, and vascular anomalies, intrauterine factors, and enteroviral infections.

COMMONLY USED CHILDHOOD INTERVENTIONS

Nonsurgical Treatment

Nonsurgical treatment of clubfoot is widely accepted as both the initial and the mainstay of treatment. The Ponseti method of serial clubfoot manipulation and casting, Achilles tenotomy, and bracing the foot in abduction has become the gold standard of clubfoot correction, with the highest reported long-term success rates. This method is indicated for the treatment of idiopathic clubfoot and is increasingly being used for the treatment of severe nonidiopathic clubfoot deformities, the complex clubfoot (as defined by Ponseti), and for recurrent deformity following previous extensive soft-tissue release.[7]

Treatment is initiated within the first few weeks of life and consists of a series of gentle manipulations of

---

Dr. Chao or an immediate family member has stock or stock options held in Abbott, Bristol-Myers Squibb, and Express Scripts. Neither Dr. Ramineni nor any immediate family member has received anything of value from or owns stock in a commercial company or institution related directly or indirectly to the subject of this chapter.

the foot, followed by the application of a long-leg cast on a weekly basis in the office setting. The cavus deformity is corrected by supination of the forefoot with direct pressure beneath the first metatarsal at the time of first manipulation and casting. Forefoot adduction and hindfoot varus are corrected simultaneously with the subsequent casts by gently abducting the forefoot in supination while applying counterpressure laterally over the head of the talus. To avoid creation of a rocker-bottom deformity, equinus is corrected only after forefoot adduction and heel varus are corrected.[8] When equinus persists after forefoot and hindfoot correction, a percutaneous Achilles tenotomy is performed under local anesthesia, followed by the application of a cast with the foot in 70° of abduction and 5° to 10° of dorsiflexion. Ponseti[8] reported that Achilles tenotomy was required in 70% of his patients. Once complete radiographic correction is achieved and the final cast is removed, the patient is fitted with a foot abduction brace to prevent recurrence of the deformity. Ponseti recommended that the brace be worn until the child is 2 to 4 years of age. Currently, many clinicians discontinue splinting once the child is able to walk independently.[9]

Kite[10] recommended correction of forefoot adduction by gently pushing the navicular onto the head of the talus with the index finger while placing the thumb laterally over the distal end of the calcaneus to act as a fulcrum. Longitudinal studies reveal a much higher incidence of surgical intervention with this technique when compared with the Ponseti technique.[11]

The nonsurgical technique developed by Bensahel (the French functional method) involves daily gentle manipulation of the foot by a physical therapist for 30 minutes, followed by taping of the foot in between sessions for the first 2 months.[12] Elastic tape is used as a splint to help maintain the correction. The frequency of treatment decreases to three times per week for 8 months. Although acceptable results have been reported by Johnston and Richards,[13] the logistics of this treatment regimen are difficult to arrange in the current healthcare environment.

Surgical Treatment

Surgery is indicated for cases of idiopathic and neurogenic clubfoot that do not respond to nonsurgical treatment and for recurrent deformities following nonsurgical treatment or initial surgical correction. Bensahel et al[14] described an "à la carte" approach to the surgical correction of the clubfoot. The authors recommended releasing the structures only as needed to obtain adequate correction of the foot. Advocates of early treatment will perform the surgery when the child is between 3 and 6 months of age, whereas advocates of late treatment prefer to wait until 9 to 12 months of age. The circumferential Cincinnati incision is often preferred when extensive soft-tissue release is planned. The medial plantar release, posterior release, and lateral release are performed through the circumferential incision. Most patients often need only the posterior release because the tight medial structures often respond to casting.

Outcomes

In 1995, Cooper and Dietz[15] reviewed 45 patients who had 71 congenital clubfeet treated using the Ponseti technique of serial manipulation, casting, Achilles tenotomy, and splinting with a Denis Browne splint. The authors found that 78% of patients had an excellent or good outcome compared with 85% of 97 individuals who did not have congenital deformity of the foot. Hertzenberg et al[16] compared 27 patients treated using the Ponseti method with 27 patients treated using traditional casting techniques. One patient in the Ponseti group required a posteromedial release compared with 91% of patients in the control group. Lehman et al[17] reported a 92% initial success rate within the first year of life.

Despite the wide variation in surgical procedures for clubfoot, various reports documented 60% to 80% excellent or good results following surgical correction.[18,19] Of the residual abnormalities that are found in the surgically corrected foot, the most prominent are weakness in the gastrocnemius-soleus complex and difficulty with push-off. Other abnormalities include some element of footdrop and persistent internal rotation deformity of the foot. Despite these abnormalities, function is generally good and compatible with normal shoe wear and full activity.

ADULT SEQUELAE
Presenting Symptoms

The adult presentation of an individual born with a clubfoot deformity varies with the type of treatment that the individual received in childhood. Historically, clubfoot is recognized as a significant foot and ankle condition in newborns and treatment is usually started shortly after birth. Sometimes, several surgical procedures are necessary to correct the deformities. Surgical correction of clubfoot, which was once popular in the 1970s and 1980s, is now less popular because of unfavorable results in the adult population with clubfoot. The most common presentation of the surgically corrected clubfoot is severe hindfoot stiffness. Other common presenting symptoms include residual deformities, pain with or without weight bearing, recurrent ankle sprains, and shoe wear problems.

Most common residual clubfoot deformities in adults are usually the result of incomplete correction by casting. Persistent midfoot cavus is usually due to failure to adequately elevate the first ray before abducting the foot at the talonavicular joint. Residual forefoot adductus and hindfoot varus can also be seen following incomplete correction. These patients place more weight on and push-off along the lateral border of the foot. These patients also usually report lateral foot pain and/or recurrent ankle sprains. Improper casting technique results in more severe deformities including rocker-bottom deformity of the midfoot due to inappropriate correction of equinus while the calcaneus remains internally rotated and locked beneath the talus. Persistent valgus hindfoot may be due to insufficient release of calcaneofibular ligament, injudicious release of the interosseous ligament of the subtalar joint resulting in subtalar instability, or posterior tibial tendon insufficiency due to excessive lengthening. These patients report weakness in toe-off and pain. Lateral impingement between the calcaneus and the fibula may also result from lateral displacement of the calcaneus and, over time, may lead to midfoot collapse. Incompetence of the spring ligament or the posterior tibial tendon may result in pes planus. Relative overpull of the tibialis anterior tendon with weak peroneus longus may result in forefoot supination and dorsal bunion.

Evaluation
Physical Examination
Physical examination begins with careful observation of the patient's gait. The nature of ground contact, the position of the heel, and the position of the toes during stance phase all should be observed. The presence of any footdrop, dynamic supination, and cock-up deformity of the great toe during swing phase should be noted. With the patient standing, the position of the hindfoot and the presence of cavus or planus should be observed.

With the patient seated, the active and passive range of motion of the ankle, subtalar, transverse tarsal, and metatarsophalangeal joints of both lower extremities are determined. The presence of equinus contracture should be assessed. The muscle function and strength of both feet and ankles should be carefully tested, with attention given to the tibialis anterior, tibialis posterior, peroneal longus and brevis, and the gastrocnemius-soleus complex. The ability to perform a single-stance heel rise should be noted. The relative position of the forefoot to the hindfoot should be determined. If a deformity is present, whether the deformity is passively correctable to a neutral plantigrade foot should be noted. The Coleman block test is used to determine the rigidity of a forefoot-driven hindfoot varus deformity. The stability of the subtalar joint and both sides of the ankle should be tested. The location of surgical scars and calluses should be noted and the patient's neurovascular status should be carefully documented.

Imaging Studies
Weight-bearing radiographs of the ankle and foot are critical in evaluating clubfoot in the adult using the angles listed in **Table 1**. The presence of metatarsus adductus should be noted on the AP view, as it may require some degree of surgical correction. The talus develops adaptive changes with age and the dome may be flattened, thereby limiting the amount of dorsiflexion at the ankle. Any degenerative changes in the foot and/or ankle need to be documented.

CT may be indicated to further evaluate bony details, especially alignment and the severity of degenerative changes. CT helps determine the alignment of the subtalar joint, hindfoot, and midfoot in patients with undercorrection or overcorrection from previous surgery. MRI helps evaluate soft-tissue structures and bone marrow for avascular changes in bony structures.

INTERVENTIONS FOR THE ADULT PATIENT
Nonsurgical Treatment
The goal of nonsurgical treatment of clubfoot in the adult is to alleviate pain and restore function. The treat-

TABLE 1 Radiographic Evaluation of Clubfoot in the Adult

Angle	Definition	Characteristics
Lateral talar–first metatarsal	Measured on the lateral view. The angle subtended by the long axes of the talus and the first metatarsal.	Normally, these lines are collinear. In the cavus foot, the apex is directed dorsally; in pes planus, the apex is directed plantarly.
Lateral talocalcaneal	Measured on the lateral view. The angle is subtended by the long axis of the talus and the plantar surface of the calcaneus.	This angle measures approximately 30°–45° in the normal foot, is decreased with hindfoot varus, and increased with hindfoot valgus.
AP talocalcaneal	Measured on the AP view.	The angle measures approximately 30°–45° in the normal foot, is decreased with hindfoot varus, and increased with hindfoot valgus.
Calcaneal pitch	Measured on the lateral view. The angle between the plantar and horizontal surfaces of the calcaneus.	This angle indicates the position of the calcaneus in stance and is elevated in hindfoot cavus.

ment needs to be individualized depending on the specific problems. Physical therapy is recommended for patients presenting with soft-tissue conditions such as a tight Achilles tendon, mild Achilles tendon contracture, mild weakness in the posterior tibial tendon, or mild tightness along other tendons or joints. If the deformities are flexible and can be passively corrected to neutral, the joints and soft-tissue structures can be better supported with customized orthotic shoe inserts, a University of California Biomechanics Laboratory (UCBL) insert, or a customized above-the-ankle brace. Mild flexible residual deformities presenting with metatarsalgia, calluses, and claw toes can be treated with a semirigid orthosis with a metatarsal pad. More severe deformities with hindfoot varus may be controlled with an articulated or solid-ankle molded ankle-foot orthosis. Often, the deformities are severe and less amenable to bracing, in which case surgical options have to be considered.

Surgical Treatment

The goal of surgical management is to achieve a plantigrade, stable foot. The surgical plan is based on the specific deformities that need to be addressed and the rigidity of those deformities. The treatment options include soft-tissue releases with or without tendon transfers, osteotomies, limited fusions, or triple arthrodesis. It is always preferable to maintain a flexible foot and to avoid fusion, if feasible.

Equinus Deformity

Most patients with residual clubfoot have persistent equinus deformity, which can be corrected with percutaneous Achilles tendon lengthening. Gastrocnemius recession may be performed for isolated gastrocnemius contracture, which is rare. More rigid equinus deformities may need a posterior ankle capsular release along with Achilles tendon lengthening. To prevent calcaneal deformity, overzealous lengthening of the Achilles tendon should be avoided. It may be necessary to release the deltoid ligament and the posterior syndesmotic ligaments if the ankle cannot be corrected adequately following posterior capsulotomy. This release will allow the talus to rotate posteriorly in the ankle mortise.

Hindfoot Varus and Forefoot Adduction

Hindfoot varus is usually associated with forefoot medial deviation and cavus. Hindfoot varus also may be secondary to plantar flexion of the first ray where the deformity is flexible and can be differentiated from a rigid deformity by using the Coleman block test. Hindfoot varus is generally rigid in clubfoot. The treatment of persistent hindfoot varus depends on the cause and the extent of the associated deformity. A Z-plasty of the posterior tibial tendon, flexor digitorum longus, and flexor hallucis longus may be required, along with medial talonavicular capsular release to correct forefoot adduction. If soft-tissue release of the foot fails, lateral column shortening will be required in the form of wedge osteotomy, either through the calcaneus, the calcaneocuboid joint, or the cuboid to achieve satisfactory alignment. Rigid hindfoot varus is corrected using a combination of a lateral closing wedge (Dwyer) osteotomy and sliding of the calcaneus. A closing wedge osteotomy alone decreases the heel height significantly, making shoe fitting difficult. Release of the plantar fascia (Steindler stripping) is often performed in conjunction with calcaneal osteotomy to decrease the height of the longitudinal arch in patients with flexible deformities. A dorsiflexion osteotomy of the first metatarsal is required to correct forefoot-driven hindfoot varus.

Hindfoot Valgus

Hindfoot valgus may result from a surgical overcorrection of clubfoot, including posterior tibial insufficiency, injudicious release of the interosseous ligament of the subtalar joint, or incomplete release of the calcaneofibular ligament. Hindfoot valgus may be associated with rigid forefoot supination. Flexible hindfoot valgus deformity can be corrected with a medial displacement osteotomy of the calcaneus. Lateral column lengthening is added to correct severe forefoot abduction. Subtalar instability with severe hindfoot valgus can be corrected using subtalar arthrodesis with an iliac crest graft wedged laterally to improve the weight-bearing axis through the subtalar joint. In severe and rigid deformities with or without degenerative arthritis, triple arthrodesis may be required.

Severe Residual Clubfoot Deformity

Limited fusion or triple arthrodesis is required to correct a severely deformed and stiff clubfoot. Fusion is indicated for degenerative arthritis involving the subtalar or calcaneocuboid joints. Triple arthrodesis can achieve a stiff, plantigrade foot in the presence of severe residual clubfoot.

EXPERT OPINION

In general, the approach to nonsurgical and surgical treatment of clubfoot in adults is similar to other types of adult-acquired foot and ankle deformities. A detailed history should be obtained and a physical examination needs to be performed. Most patients complain of stiffness, difficulty walking on uneven surfaces, and finding shoes that fit comfortably. Physical examination of the foot and ankle should be performed to assess the range of motion of the ankle, subtalar, transverse tarsal, and metatarsophalangeal joints. It is important to determine whether the deformity is fixed or flexible. Most patients with clubfoot have rigid deformities. For patients who have flexible deformities, muscle strength testing is especially important to determine whether tendon transfer is feasible to restore function.

Weight-bearing radiographs of the foot and ankle are necessary to assess alignment. Weight-bearing radiographs of the ankle, tibia and fibula, and knee are sometimes necessary to assess the relationship between any foot and ankle deformity and the knee joint. CT helps evaluate the condition and the alignment of the midfoot, hindfoot, and ankle joint. MRI and ultrasonography (static and dynamic) help evaluate the soft-tissue structures as well as tendon function.

Nonsurgical treatment includes bracing and off-loading the deformity. Surgery is indicated for patients in whom nonsurgical treatment has failed. If the deformity is flexible and passively correctable to neutral and the muscle strength is normal, then correction of the deformity can be achieved through osteotomies and tendon transfer. Because most adults with a history of clubfoot present with rigid deformities and degenerative changes in the foot and ankle joints, arthrodesis and osteotomy are more commonly performed to create a plantigrade, functional foot.

CONCLUSION

To understand the treatment of clubfoot deformity in an adult, it is necessary to understand the pathophysiology of the deformity. By understanding any previous treatment, the residual deformity, and the patient's problems at presentation, the surgeon can devise the appropriate treatment recommendation. The goal of the treatment is to eliminate pain and, if necessary, to correct the deformity with or without surgery.

REFERENCES

1. Wynne-Davies R: Family studies and the cause of congenital clubfoot: Talipes equinovarus, talipes calcaneovalgus, and metatarsus varus. *J Bone Joint Surg Br* 1964;46:445-463.
2. Bakalis S, Sairam S, Homfray T, Harrington K, Nicolaides K, Thilaganathan B: Outcome of antenatally

diagnosed talipes equinovarus in an unselected obstetric population. *Ultrasound Obstet Gynecol* 2002;20(3): 226-229.

3. Gordon N: Arthrogryposis multiplex congenita. *Brain Dev* 1998;20(7):507-511.

4. Gurnett CA, Boehm S, Connolly A, Reimschisel T, Dobbs MB: Impact of congenital talipes equinovarus etiology on treatment outcomes. *Dev Med Child Neurol* 2008;50(7):498-502.

5. Shimizu N, Hamada S, Mitta M, Hiroshima K, Ono K: Etiological considerations of congenital clubfoot deformity, in Tachdjian MO, Simons G, eds: *The Clubfoot: The Present and a View of the Future.* New York, NY, Springer, 1993, pp 31-38.

6. Lochmiller C, Johnston D, Scott A, Risman M, Hecht JT: Genetic epidemiology study of idiopathic talipes equinovarus. *Am J Med Genet* 1998;79(2):90-96.

7. Ponseti IV, Zhivkov M, Davis N, Sinclair M, Dobbs MB, Morcuende JA: Treatment of the complex idiopathic clubfoot. *Clin Orthop Relat Res* 2006(451):171-176.

8. Ponseti IV: Treatment of congenital club foot. *J Bone Joint Surg Am* 1992;74(3):448-454.

9. Cummings RJ, Davidson RS, Armstrong PF, Lehman WB: Congenital clubfoot. *J Bone Joint Surg Am* 2002; 84-A(2):290-308.

10. Kite JH: *The Clubfoot.* New York, NY, Grune and Stratton, 1964.

11. Sud A, Tiwari A, Sharma D, Kapoor S: Ponseti's vs. Kite's method in the treatment of clubfoot—a prospective randomised study. *Int Orthop* 2008;32(3):409-413.

12. Bensahel H, Guillaume A, Czukonyi Z, Desgrippes Y: Results of physical therapy for idiopathic clubfoot: A long-term follow-up study. *J Pediatr Orthop* 1990;10(2):189-192.

13. Johnston W, Richards BS: Non-operative treatment of clubfoot-the French technique, in *Proceedings of the Pediatric Orthopaedic Society of North America, Annual Meeting.* Lake Buena Vista, FL, May 15-19, 1999, p 25.

14. Bensahel H, Csukonyi Z, Desgrippes Y, Chaumien JP: Surgery in residual clubfoot: One-stage medioposterior release "à la carte". *J Pediatr Orthop* 1987;7(2):145-148.

15. Cooper DM, Dietz FR: Treatment of idiopathic clubfoot: A thirty-year follow-up note. *J Bone Joint Surg Am* 1995;77(10):1477-1489.

16. Herzenberg JE, Radler C, Bor N: Ponseti versus traditional methods of casting for idiopathic clubfoot. *J Pediatr Orthop* 2002;22(4):517-521.

17. Lehman WB, Mohaideen A, Madan S, et al: A method for the early evaluation of the Ponseti (Iowa) technique for the treatment of idiopathic clubfoot. *J Pediatr Orthop B* 2003;12(2):133-140.

18. Cohen-Sobel E, Caselli M, Giorgini R, Giorgini T, Stummer S: Long-term follow-up of clubfoot surgery: Analysis of 44 patients. *J Foot Ankle Surg* 1993;32(4):411-423.

19. Turco VJ: Resistant congenital club foot—one-stage posteromedial release with internal fixation: A follow-up report of a fifteen-year experience. *J Bone Joint Surg Am* 1979;61(6A):805-814.

CHAPTER *6*

TARSAL COALITION

WEN CHAO, MD

SATHEESH KUMAR RAMINENI, MD

INTRODUCTION

A tarsal coalition is a fibrous, cartilaginous, or bony connection of two or more bones of the hindfoot or midfoot. Tarsal coalition is associated with rigid pes planus, also called rigid flatfoot, and peroneal muscle spasm. The incidence of this condition occurs in fewer than 1% of the population.[1] The most common symptomatic tarsal coalitions are of the calcaneonavicular joint and the middle facet of the talocalcaneal joint;[2] these account for 90% of all tarsal coalitions[1] and are bilateral in 50% to 60% of cases. Other coalitions, including those of the talonavicular, calcaneocuboid, naviculocuboid, and naviculocuneiform joints, are rare.

A coalition is thought to be a failure of primitive mesenchyme to segment and produce a normal peritalar joint complex.[2] Some authors have suggested a hereditary tendency for tarsal coalition; Leonard[3] confirmed an autosomal pattern of inheritance.

The possible etiologies for symptomatic tarsal coalition include stress reaction or stress fracture that occurs during progressive ossification and limited hindfoot mobility with altered biomechanics that results in increased stress across the involved joints. Calcaneonavicular coalition usually becomes symptomatic in patients who are 8 to 14 years of age, when the ossification of the coalition occurs. Talocalcaneal coalition rarely becomes symptomatic in patients younger than 12 years. The coalition may be fibrous (syndesmosis), cartilaginous (synchondrosis), or bony (synostosis). Patients with talocalcaneal coalition present with vague dorsolateral foot pain, difficulty walking on uneven surfaces, and loss of the longitudinal arch. Talocalcaneal coalition is frequently associated with recurrent ankle sprains. Physical examination may reveal severe, progressive pes planus deformity. The classic finding is marked reduction or complete absence of subtalar motion. When the patient rises to the balls of the feet, the hindfoot does not invert to its normal varus position. Peroneal muscle spasm often is present with talocalcaneal coalition.

Calcaneonavicular coalition is best seen on a 45° lateral oblique radiograph of the foot, with the abnormal coalition extending from the anterior process of the calcaneus just lateral to the anterior facet dorsally and to the lateral and dorsolateral extra-articular surfaces of the navicular medially. Other radiographic signs include the anteater nose sign, the C sign, and beaking of the talar head. Talocalcaneal coalition can be seen on a 45° axial view of the calcaneus (Harris Beath view). Other radiographic findings include the loss of a normal middle facet of the talocalcaneal joint, broadening or rounding of the lateral talar process, talar head beaking, and loss of the medial subtalar joint space. A weight-bearing AP view of the ankle should be obtained in all cases of suspected tarsal coalition. A ball-and-socket ankle may be seen in cases of long-standing tarsal coalition.[4]

Triphasic bone scanning helps identify the cause of foot pain in the patient with an atypical history for subtalar coalition.[5] Triphasic bone scanning is also a good screening tool with high sensitivity to help diagnose foot and ankle pathology. CT is the best imaging method for the assessment of subtalar coalition,[6] although MRI was shown recently to be almost as good as CT.[7] When other bony or soft-tissue lesions of the hindfoot or midfoot need to be considered in the differential diagnosis, MRI is indicated. MRI also helps identify the type of coalition (fibrous, cartilaginous, or bony). Laboratory workup including complete blood count with differential, erythrocyte sedimentation rate, C-reactive protein, rheumatoid factor, and antinuclear antibody are recommended to rule out infection or other inflammatory processes.

NATURAL HISTORY

Approximately 25% of individuals with tarsal coalition develop symptoms.[3] The onset of pain coincides with the progression of ossification, which usually occurs between 8 and 12 years of age with calcaneonavicular coalition and between 12 and 16 years of age with talocalcaneal coalition. As the coalition becomes symptomatic, valgus deformity of the hindfoot progresses, the longitudinal arch flattens, and subtalar motion is restricted.[8]

TREATMENT

The goal of treatment is relief of pain and restoration of motion. Nonsurgical treatment is the first line of management of symptomatic tarsal coalition.[2,6,9] Activity modification, arch supports, medial heel wedges, and University of California Biomechanics Laboratory (UCBL) orthoses may help individuals with mild symptoms. Cast immobilization for 4 to 6 weeks may help individuals with severe symptoms.

Surgical treatment is indicated if symptoms continue despite extensive nonsurgical treatment. Surgical options include excision with or without osteotomy and arthrodesis. Some reports suggest that excision of the coalition and some form of interposition using the extensor digitorum brevis (EDB) muscle or fat is the best surgical treatment for calcaneonavicular resection. Good to excellent results of 70% to 100% were reported at

11- to 23-year follow-up.[10-18] Talar head beaking is no longer considered a contraindication for resection. Poor results were associated with incomplete resection and the presence of degenerative changes in the hindfoot joints. Significant degenerative changes in the talonavicular and calcaneocuboid joints are contraindications to surgical excision. If degenerative changes of the hindfoot joints exist, then arthrodesis of the arthritic joints is indicated.

Indications for talocalcaneal resection are less clear and more complicated. Various factors have been described as important predictors of outcome and to determine the appropriate surgical intervention. These factors include the age of the patient, the size and type of the coalition, the degree of hindfoot valgus, and the presence of degenerative changes within the surrounding joints. If a patient has a talocalcaneal coalition that does not respond to nonsurgical treatment in the absence of degenerative changes in the adjacent joints, the current consensus on treatment is coalition excision. A split portion of flexor hallucis longus tendon, fat, and bone wax all have been used as interposition material.[15-20] In general, the outcome of surgical treatment of talocalcaneal coalition is less favorable than outcomes for calcaneonavicular resection. The factors associated with poor prognosis include greater degrees of heel valgus, larger coalition size, increasing age, and the presence of advanced degenerative changes.[9,12,16,17,21] Triple arthrodesis is indicated for the salvage of failed resection.[12]

ADULT SEQUELAE
Presenting Symptoms

Symptomatic talocalcaneal and calcaneonavicular coalitions occur with almost equal frequency in adults and children. Adult patients with tarsal coalition may present with dorsolateral hindfoot pain in the sinus tarsi region, vague ankle and hindfoot pain, recurrent ankle sprains, lateral ankle instability, and rigid, painful pes planus.[22-25] Symptoms may be the result of associated degenerative changes in the hindfoot articulations. Adult patients with tarsal coalition rarely present with peroneal spasm.[22] Adult patients with talocalcaneal coalition may present with symptoms consistent with tarsal tunnel syndrome because the coalition is near the posterior tibial nerve. Patients who present with other conditions such as posterior tibial tendon dysfunction may be symptomatic for tarsal coalition.

Evaluation
Physical Examination
The physical examination should be performed with the patient standing and sitting. Gait should be analyzed, with emphasis placed on stance-phase biomechanics. The standing examination should include assessment of the hindfoot posture (neutral, valgus, varus), evaluation of the longitudinal arch, and the single-limb heel rise. Most adults with tarsal coalition present with a neutral heel. Valgus posture is the second most common symptom, and rarely, patients may present with varus hindfoot. The sitting examination should include assessment of the range of motion of the ankle, subtalar, and transverse tarsal joints, muscle strength grade and peroneal spasm, eliciting tenderness to palpation at the middle facet of the talocalcaneal joint or at the calcaneonavicular joint, and determination of lateral ankle instability. A classic, consistent finding is limited or complete loss of subtalar joint motion compared with the unaffected extremity that is more pronounced with talocalcaneal coalition.

Imaging Studies
Plain radiographs of the foot and ankle should be obtained with the patient standing. A Harris Beath view should be obtained for the patient with suspected talocalcaneal coalition. A 45° lateral oblique view of the foot helps identify calcaneonavicular coalition. The radiographic signs, as discussed earlier, are the same in children and adolescents with calcaneonavicular and talocalcaneal coalition, the two most common types. Bone scanning helps identify the cause of pain in patients who have vague and atypical pain at presentation. CT and MRI are indicated if radiography is inconclusive. These imaging studies help identify the nature of coalition, exclude associated pathology, and identify the presence of degenerative changes in the surrounding articulations.

INTERVENTIONS FOR THE ADULT PATIENT
Literature Review
Few reports discuss tarsal coalition in the adult population. In 1974, Rankin and Baker[25] reported on 17 adults in basic military training (age range, 17 to 22 years) with radiographic evidence of tarsal coalition and found 9 instances of talocalcaneal coalition and 5 instances of calcaneonavicular coalition. All patients had rigid pes planus with diminished subtalar motion. Patients were treated nonsurgically with activity modification. No follow-up or clinical outcomes were mentioned in the report.

In 1988, Percy and Mann[24] reported on 9 patients (age range, 15 to 49 years) with 13 tarsal coalitions. All patients presented with painful pes planus and had talocalcaneal coalition with limited subtalar motion. Six patients were treated nonsurgically with rest, NSAIDs, orthotic use, and custom shoe modification and/or casting; two patients underwent triple arthrodesis; and one patient underwent a Grice procedure.

Cohen et al[22] reported on 12 adult patients (age range, 19 to 48 years) with calcaneonavicular coalition in 13 symptomatic feet. Nonsurgical treatment failed in all patients. Preoperatively, 10 feet had radiographic evidence of degenerative arthritis and 7 feet had evidence of talar head beaking. All patients underwent calcaneonavicular resection. At a mean postoperative follow-up of 36 months, eight patients had subjective relief of symptoms. Two patients with symptomatic coalition underwent subsequent hindfoot arthrodesis.

Varner and Michelson[23] reported on tarsal coalition in 21 symptomatic feet in adults (age range, 16 to 81 years). Nonsurgical treatment was successful in most patients. Subtalar fusion was performed in four feet and coalition resection in one foot.

Scott and Tuten[26] reported the results of calcaneonavicular coalition resection with EDB interposition in seven adult patients (mean age, 41 years) on eight symptomatic feet who had no radiographic evidence of degenerative arthritis. All patients had a satisfactory outcome at a mean follow-up of 56.5 months.

Philbin et al[27] reported on the results of talocalcaneal coalition resection in seven patients (age range, 15 to 56 years), with a mean follow-up of 17.4 months. Resection was successful in six patients, one of whom underwent subtalar arthrodesis 1 year after the index procedure. The authors concluded that a higher cartilage content in the coalition correlated with a better outcome.

Nonsurgical Treatment
Nonsurgical treatment is the first line of management of symptomatic tarsal coalition. Activity modification,

arch supports, medial heel wedges, and UCBL orthoses may help individuals with mild symptoms. Cast immobilization for 4 to 6 weeks may help individuals with severe symptoms.

Surgical Treatment

If extensive nonsurgical treatment fails in symptomatic tarsal coalition, surgical treatment is indicated. If the coalition is relatively small and the involved joints have minimal degenerative changes, then coalition excision with or without osteotomy is indicated to correct the deformity. If moderate to significant degenerative changes and/or deformities are present, then osteotomy to correct the deformities and arthrodesis of the degenerative joints are indicated. Current evidence suggests that coalition excision with EDB interposition is the best surgical treatment of calcaneonavicular coalition. Talar head beaking is no longer considered a contraindication for resection. Poor results were associated with incomplete resection and the presence of degenerative changes in the hindfoot joints.[10,12,17,28,29] Substantial degenerative changes in the talonavicular and calcaneocuboid joints are contraindications to surgical excision.

EXPERT OPINION

Various factors have been described as important in predicting outcomes and determining the appropriate surgical intervention for talocalcaneal resection, including patient age, the size and composition of the coalition, the degree of hindfoot valgus, and the presence of degenerative changes within the surrounding joints. For patients with talocalcaneal coalition in whom nonsurgical treatment has failed, the consensus on current treatment is coalition excision in the absence of degenerative changes in the adjacent joints with or without interposition of a split portion of the flexor hallucis longus tendon or interposition with fat or bone wax. Most adults who undergo surgery for symptomatic talocalcaneal coalition experience degenerative changes in the subtalar and surrounding joints. Therefore, fusion of the degenerative joints is preformed more frequently than excision of the talocalcaneal coalition. The outcomes for talocalcaneal resection are less favorable than those for calcaneonavicular resection. Poor prognosis is associated with greater degrees of heel valgus, larger coalition size, the existence of a bony coalition, increasing patient age, and the presence of advanced degenerative changes. Subtalar arthrodesis is used more often than triple arthrodesis for the salvage of failed resection.

CONCLUSION

The presentation of tarsal coalition in adults is similar to that in the younger population. Most patients complain of painful, rigid pes planus. The physical examination and diagnostic studies used to determine the diagnosis are also similar. If a patient's nonsurgical treatment fails, surgery is indicated. Surgical treatment depends on the degree of degenerative changes in the affected and surrounding joints.

REFERENCES

1. Stormont DM, Peterson HA: The relative incidence of tarsal coalition. *Clin Orthop Relat Res* 1983(181):28-36.
2. Harris R, Beath T: Etiology of peroneal spastic flatfoot. *J Bone Joint Surg Br* 1948;30:624-634.
3. Leonard MA: The inheritance of tarsal coalition and its relationship to spastic flat foot. *J Bone Joint Surg Br* 1974;56-B(3):520-526.
4. Conway JJ, Cowell HR: Tarsal coalition: Clinical significance and roentgenographic demonstration. *Radiology* 1969;92(4):799-811.
5. Deutsch AL, Resnick D, Campbell G: Computed tomography and bone scintigraphy in the evaluation of tarsal coalition. *Radiology* 1982;144(1):137-140.
6. Herzenberg JE, Goldner JL, Martinez S, Silverman PM: Computerized tomography of talocalcaneal tarsal coalition: A clinical and anatomic study. *Foot Ankle* 1986;6(6):273-288.
7. Emery KH, Bisset GS III, Johnson ND, Nunan PJ: Tarsal coalition: A blinded comparison of MRI and CT. *Pediatr Radiol* 1998;28(8):612-616.
8. Kasser JR: Congenital deformities and malformation of the foot (natural history through treatment), in Morrissy RT, Weinstein SL, eds: *Lovell and Winter's Pediatric Orthopaedics*, ed 6. Philadelphia, PA, Lippincott Williams & Wilkins, 2006, vol 2, pp 1262-1277.
9. Cowell HR: Diagnosis and management of peroneal spastic flatfoot. *Instr Course Lect* 1975;24:94-103.
10. Andreasen E: Calcaneo-navicular coalition: Late results of resection. *Acta Orthop Scand* 1968;39(3):424-432.
11. Chambers RB, Cook TM, Cowell HR: Surgical reconstruction for calcaneonavicular coalition: Evaluation of

function and gait. *J Bone Joint Surg Am* 1982;64(6): 829-836.

12. Swiontkowski MF, Scranton PE, Hansen S: Tarsal coalitions: Long-term results of surgical treatment. *J Pediatr Orthop* 1983;3(3):287-292.

13. Gonzalez P, Kumar SJ: Calcaneonavicular coalition treated by resection and interposition of the extensor digitorum brevis muscle. *J Bone Joint Surg Am* 1990;72(1):71-77.

14. Moyes ST, Crawfurd EJ, Aichroth PM: The interposition of extensor digitorum brevis in the resection of calcaneonavicular bars. *J Pediatr Orthop* 1994;14(3):387-388.

15. Olney BW, Asher MA: Excision of symptomatic coalition of the middle facet of the talocalcaneal joint. *J Bone Joint Surg Am* 1987;69(4):539-544.

16. Kumar SJ, Guille JT, Lee MS, Couto JC: Osseous and non-osseous coalition of the middle facet of the talocalcaneal joint. *J Bone Joint Surg Am* 1992;74(4):529-535.

17. Wilde PH, Torode IP, Dickens DR, Cole WG: Resection for symptomatic talocalcaneal coalition. *J Bone Joint Surg Br* 1994;76(5):797-801.

18. McCormack TJ, Olney B, Asher M: Talocalcaneal coalition resection: A 10-year follow-up. *J Pediatr Orthop* 1997;17(1):13-15.

19. Kitaoka HB, Wikenheiser MA, Shaughnessy WJ, An KN: Gait abnormalities following resection of talocalcaneal coalition. *J Bone Joint Surg Am* 1997;79(3):369-374.

20. Raikin S, Cooperman DR, Thompson GH: Interposition of the split flexor hallucis longus tendon after resection of a coalition of the middle facet of the talocalcaneal joint. *J Bone Joint Surg Am* 1999;81(1):11-19.

21. Luhmann SJ, Schoenecker PL: Symptomatic talocalcaneal coalition resection: Indications and results. *J Pediatr Orthop* 1998;18(6):748-754.

22. Cohen BE, Davis WH, Anderson RB: Success of calcaneonavicular coalition resection in the adult population. *Foot Ankle Int* 1996;17(9):569-572.

23. Varner KE, Michelson JD: Tarsal coalition in adults. *Foot Ankle Int* 2000;21(8):669-672.

24. Percy EC, Mann DL: Tarsal coalition: A review of the literature and presentation of 13 cases. *Foot Ankle* 1988;9(1):40-44.

25. Rankin EA, Baker GI: Rigid flatfoot in the young adult. *Clin Orthop Relat Res* 1974(104):244-248.

26. Scott AT, Tuten HR: Calcaneonavicular coalition resection with extensor digitorum brevis interposition in adults. *Foot Ankle Int* 2007;28(8):890-895.

27. Philbin TM, Homan B, Hill K, Berlet G: Results of resection for middle facet tarsal coalitions in adults. *Foot Ankle Spec* 2008;1(6):344-349.

28. Takakura Y, Sugimoto K, Tanaka Y, Tamai S: Symptomatic talocalcaneal coalition: Its clinical significance and treatment. *Clin Orthop Relat Res* 1991;(269):249-256.

29. Scranton PE Jr: Treatment of symptomatic talocalcaneal coalition. *J Bone Joint Surg Am* 1987;69(4):533-539.

CHAPTER 7

UPPER EXTREMITY CONDITIONS

JOSHUA M. ABZUG, MD
SCOTT H. KOZIN, MD

INTRODUCTION

Most adult sequelae that involve the upper extremity are the result of a childhood elbow injury. The most common pediatric injuries with potential adverse sequelae in adulthood are supracondylar fractures of the distal humerus, Monteggia fracture-dislocations of the elbow, and lateral condyle fractures of the humerus.

SUPRACONDYLAR FRACTURES

Incidence of Pediatric Condition

Supracondylar fractures are the most common elbow fractures in children, with a peak incidence between 5 and 7 years of age.[1-3] Depending on the severity of the injury, fractures are treated using casting, closed reduction and percutaneous pinning, or open reduction and internal fixation. Regardless of the treatment method, coronal and/or sagittal malalignment of the fracture may result. Coronal malalignment is expressed as cubitus varus or cubitus valgus. Cubitus varus is more apparent clinically and occurs more commonly than cubitus valgus. Cubitus varus was initially thought to occur as a result of unequal growth of the distal humerus;[4,5] however, subsequent studies indicated that varus deformity is a result of varus reduction of the fracture.[6] Cubitus varus can be prevented by anatomic reduction of the fracture. Follow-up using serial radiographs is necessary

to detect early loss of reduction, which can be treated with repeat reduction. Sagittal malalignment results from incomplete fracture reduction that usually places the distal humerus fragment in extension with clinical loss of elbow flexion (**Figure 1**).

Commonly Used Childhood Interventions

In the past, isolated cubitus varus was considered primarily a cosmetic problem. More recent reports have demonstrated that patients with cubitus varus are predisposed to repeat fracture,[7] pain, and tardy posterolateral rotatory instability.[8] Spinner et al[8] reported on a series of five patients with cubitus varus in whom snapping of the medial triceps tendon and the ulnar nerve over the medial epicondyle developed. The authors treated this group of patients with valgus osteotomy of the distal humerus, with lateral transposition or partial excision of the snapping medial triceps, or a combination of both. In addition, the ulnar nerve may require decompression or transposition at the time of valgus osteotomy.[8]

Takahara et al[7] reported on a series of nine children with cubitus varus secondary to supracondylar fracture who sustained a second fracture of the distal humerus. The second fracture was usually a lateral condylar fracture, although other fracture types have been reported (**Figure 2**).

FIGURE 1

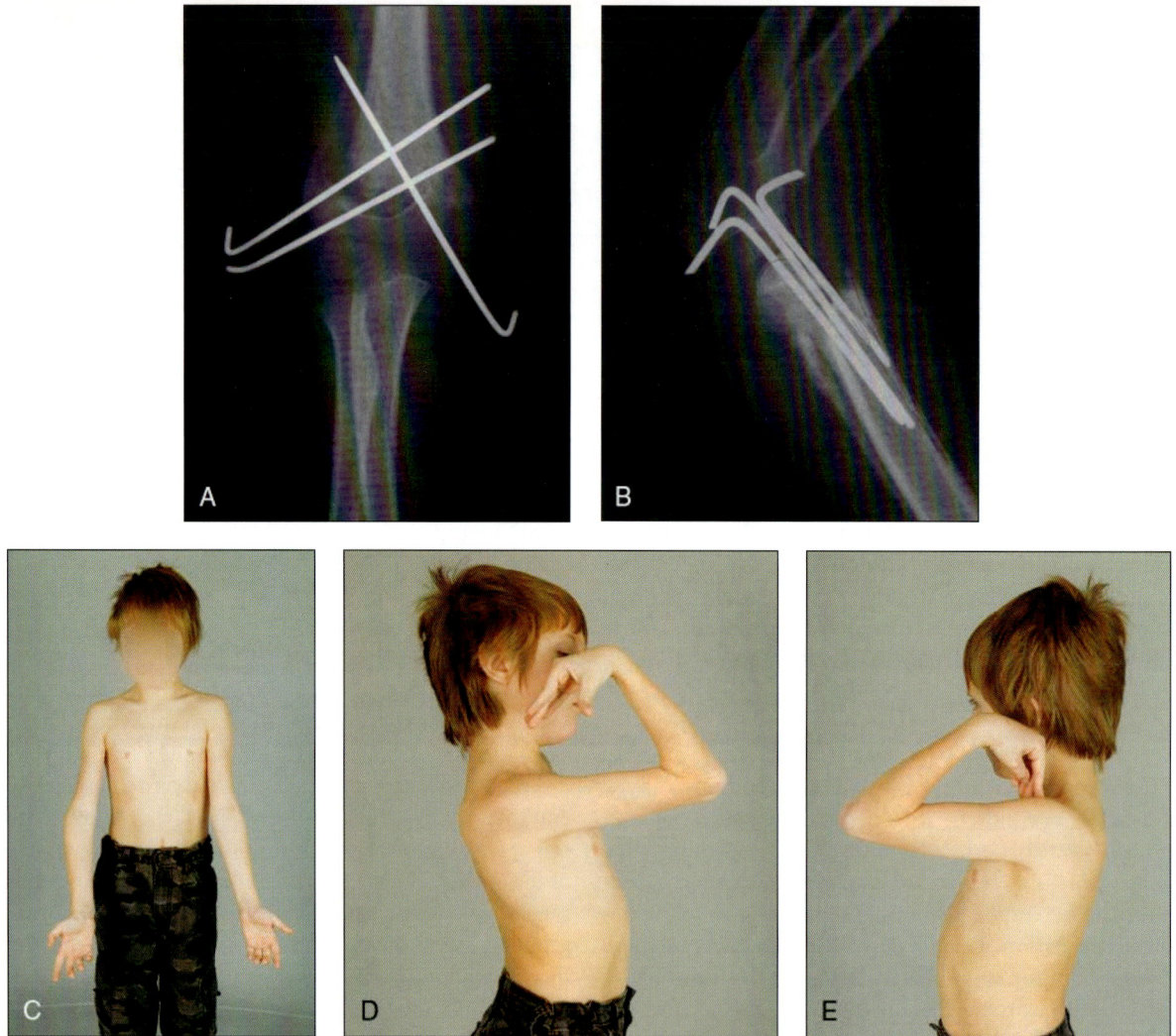

Images of a 10-year-old boy with sagittal and coronal malalignment following pin fixation of a right supracondylar fracture. **A,** AP radiograph shows pin fixation with varus alignment. **B,** Lateral radiograph shows extension of the distal fragment. Clinical photographs show right cubitus varus (**C**), deficient elbow flexion from supracondylar malunion (**D**), and contralateral elbow with full flexion (**E**). (Courtesy of Shriners Hospitals for Children, Philadelphia, PA.)

Abe et al[9] were the first to report on recurrent posterolateral dislocation of the radial head in association with cubitus varus in four patients (**Figure 3**). The dislocations occurred when the forearm was supinated and were reduced when the forearm was pronated. All patients were treated with supracondylar valgus osteotomy of the distal humerus with imbrication of the lateral ligament complex. The posterolateral elbow instability resolved in all patients.[9]

Adult Sequelae

O'Driscoll et al[10] reported on 24 patients with tardy posterolateral rotatory instability of the elbow in association with cubitus varus. In 22 patients, the cubitus

FIGURE 2

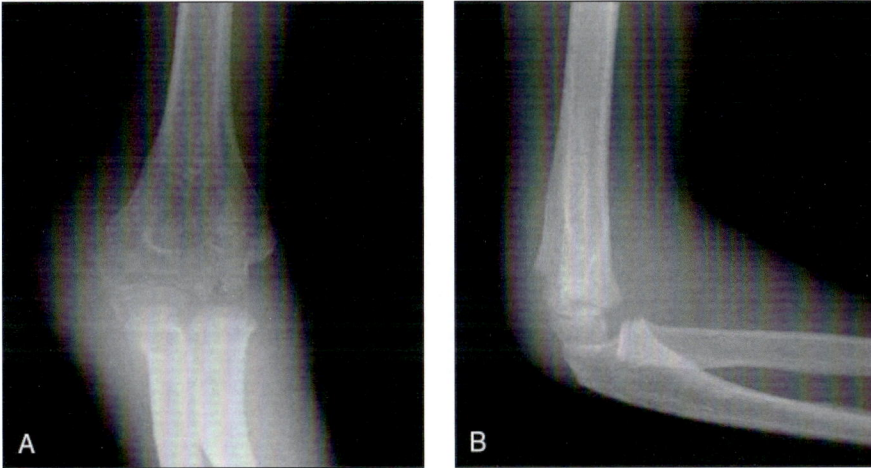

Radiographs of the elbow of a 9-year-old girl with history of a right elbow varus malunion of a supracondylar fracture. AP (**A**) and lateral (**B**) views obtained after a fall demonstrate a second elbow fracture involving the lateral condyle. (Courtesy of Shriners Hospitals for Children, Philadelphia, PA.)

varus deformity was the result of fracture malalignment; in 2 patients, the deformity was the result of congenital elbow anomalies. All patients presented 2 to 3 decades after the onset of the deformity with reports of lateral elbow pain and recurrent elbow instability. Most patients were treated with corrective osteotomy of the distal humerus and concomitant ligament reconstruction. At a mean of 3 years postoperatively, 19 of the 22 patients had results rated as good or excellent, with no recurrent instability. The authors postulated that cubitus varus caused medial displacement of the mechanical axis of the elbow and altered the force vector of the triceps. Repetitive torque in external rotation applied to the ulna attenuated the lateral collateral ligament complex, resulting in posterolateral rotatory instability.[10] These clinical observations are supported by biomechanical cadaver studies that revealed increased strain in the ulnar lateral collateral ligament complex following surgically created cubitus varus.[11]

Interventions for the Adult Patient

Cubitus varus deformity is corrected by performing osteotomy of the distal humerus. Multiple techniques have been described, including lateral closing wedge, medial opening wedge, step-cut translation, and dome osteotomies. The techniques are similar in adults and children. In adults, rigid fixation is preferred to allow early mobilization and union. In contrast, Kirschner wire (K-wire) fixation of open growth plates is pre-

FIGURE 3

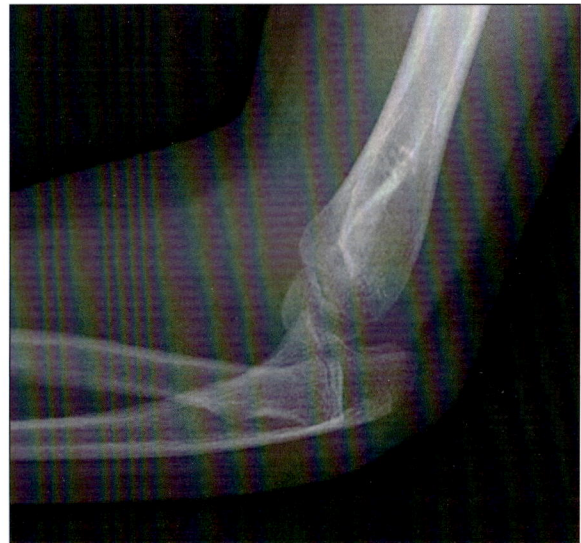

Lateral radiograph of an elbow with recurrent posterolateral instability and radial head dislocation in association with cubitus varus. (Courtesy of Shriners Hospitals for Children, Philadelphia, PA.)

ferred to avoid physeal injury because nonunion is rare and stiffness is uncommon. The dome osteotomy technique[12,13] is further discussed later in this chapter.

French[14] originally described the lateral closing wedge osteotomy in 1959; Bellemore et al[15] reported clinical results in 1984. The French technique uses a postero-

FIGURE 4

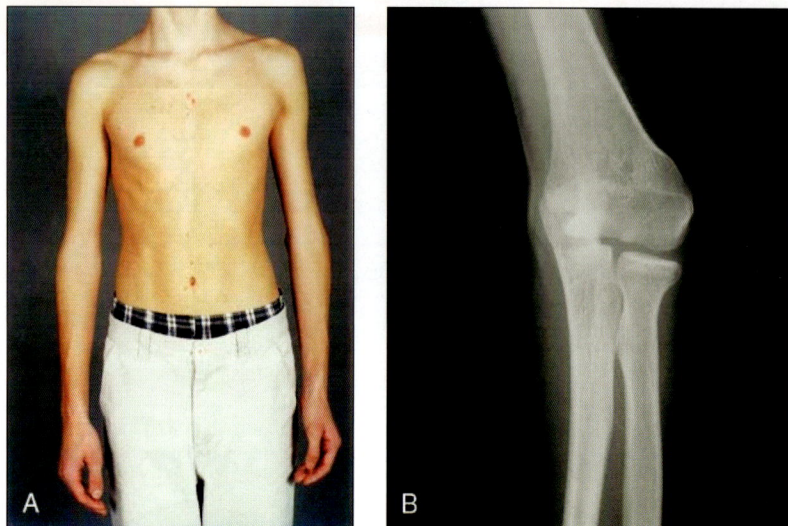

Images of a 16-year-old adolescent boy with left elbow cubitus varus. **A,** Photograph demonstrates varus alignment. **B,** AP radiograph shows reversal of carrying angle. (Courtesy of Shriners Hospitals for Children, Philadelphia, PA.)

lateral incision at the distal humerus with detachment and proximal retraction of the lateral third of the triceps tendon. An incomplete laterally based closing wedge osteotomy is created by sparing the medial cortex. Osteoclasis of the medial cortex preserves the periosteum and carefully avoids the ulnar nerve. The osteotomy is closed and the forearm is supinated to measure the carrying angle of the elbow and to compare it with the carrying angle of the opposite elbow. The osteotomy is stabilized using either plate fixation or a two-screw tension band technique. After 3 weeks of immobilization, active range of motion is initiated. Bellemore et al[15] reported good or excellent results in 23 of 27 patients treated using the French technique.

Cubitus varus or cubitus valgus deformity also may be corrected using a step-cut translation osteotomy.[16] A triangular template is fashioned preoperatively to gauge the amount of correction necessary. With the patient supine to assess the carrying angle, a posterior approach via a longitudinal midline incision is used to access the distal humerus. The ulnar nerve is identified and transposed in symptomatic patients who have numbness/tingling in the small and ring fingers. The triceps tendon is split longitudinally to expose the olecranon fossa. The template is applied 1 cm proximal to the olecranon fossa. The triangular piece of bone is removed using a saw and the distal fragment is rotated into the apex of the triangle. Additional correction can be achieved with in-

ternal rotation of the distal fragment. For cubitus varus correction, the apex of the triangle can be shifted in a medial direction to decrease the lateral prominence. Provisional fixation is achieved with K-wires and definite fixation is obtained with a Y-shaped stainless steel plate. The patient's arm is immobilized in 90° of elbow flexion and neutral forearm rotation for 3 weeks, after which active motion is started.[16]

Cubitus valgus also may be corrected using a step-cut translation osteotomy. In this case, the apex of the triangle can be shifted in a lateral direction to decrease any medial prominence. When a flexion or extension sagittal deformity is also present, a small wedge of bone can be removed from the posterior or anterior cortex of the proximal fragment to restore sagittal alignment.

Kim et al[16] performed a step-cut translation osteotomy in 32 patients and reported 26 excellent results and 6 good results. The correction of the humerus-elbow-wrist angle was 26.0° in patients with cubitus varus and 27.6° in patients with cubitus valgus. Six patients had preoperative tardy ulnar nerve palsy with complete resolution of symptoms within 1 year.[16]

Expert Opinion

Cubitus varus (**Figure 4**) is corrected with an osteotomy of the distal humerus. The authors of this chapter prefer a lateral closing wedge osteotomy (**Figure 5**) for the following reasons:[1] the technique is straightforward,[2]

FIGURE 5

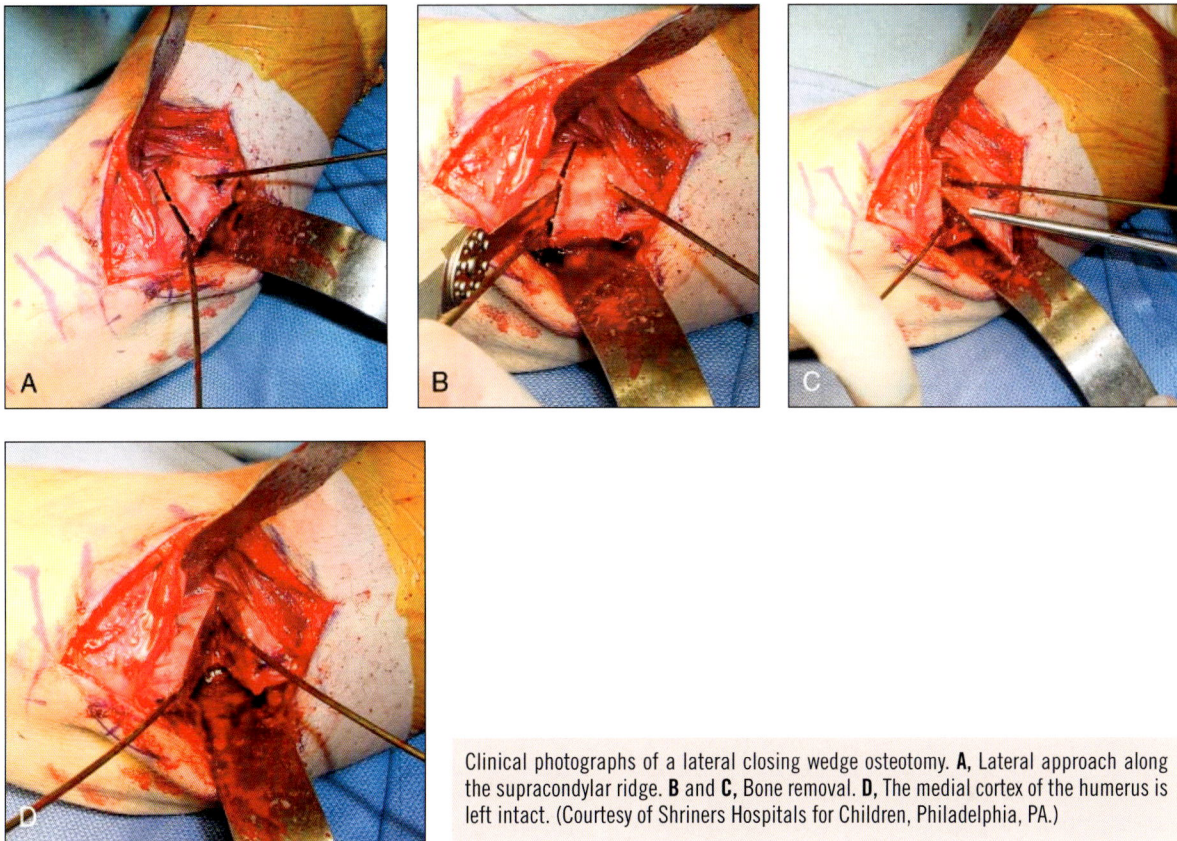

Clinical photographs of a lateral closing wedge osteotomy. **A,** Lateral approach along the supracondylar ridge. **B** and **C,** Bone removal. **D,** The medial cortex of the humerus is left intact. (Courtesy of Shriners Hospitals for Children, Philadelphia, PA.)

union is reliably achieved,[3] the lateral prominence is asymptomatic and unrecognized,[4] and the complication rate is lower than that of more complex osteotomies.[12] For treatment of moderate varus deformity of the elbow, a lateral approach along the supracondylar ridge is used. The distal humerus is exposed by elevating the biceps brachialis and the triceps. Reverse or malleable retractors are inserted across the humerus. A 0.062-inch K-wire is placed parallel to the distal humeral joint and superior to the olecranon fossa. A second 0.062-inch K-wire is placed perpendicular to the humeral shaft to determine the extent of the lateral wedge (**Figure 5, A**). Fluoroscopic evaluation ensures wire position. A bone wedge is removed between the K-wires using an oscillating saw, leaving the medial cortex of the humerus intact (**Figure 5, B** and **C**). Two additional percutaneous 0.062-inch K-wires are inserted through the lateral epicondyle and are visualized at the level of the osteotomy.

The medial cortex is cracked by applying a valgus moment to the distal humerus (**Figure 5, D**). Provisional fixation of the osteotomy is accomplished by advancing the percutaneous K-wires into the proximal fragment. Adequate correction is assessed using clinical and fluoroscopic evaluation. The percutaneous K-wires may be used as definitive fixation in the young child with open growth plates. Stable fixation is required in the adolescent and the adult using internal plate-and-screw fixation.

In patients with severe cubitus varus, a closing wedge osteotomy of the distal humerus produces a pronounced lateral elbow prominence. To minimize the prominence, the laterally based wedge can be oriented obliquely rather than parallel to the joint surface. In addition, the distal fragment can be translated in a medial direction. This procedure requires a supplemental medial incision to allow safe medial translation of the distal fragment (**Figure 6**). A long posterior incision that allows access to both sides of the elbow also can be used. When lateral and medial incisions or a posterior approach is used, rigid fixation may be obtained via dual fixation using a medial plate and a posterolateral plate. A different osteotomy configuration can also minimize any lateral prominence; the authors of this chapter prefer a dome

osteotomy via a posterior approach with elevation of the triceps (**Figure 7**).

MONTEGGIA FRACTURE-DISLOCATION

In a Monteggia fracture-dislocation, the ulnar fracture is usually recognized and reduced; however, the dislocation of the radial head may be overlooked and remain untreated. This oversight leads to a subacute or chronic dislocation of the radiocapitellar joint. The patient may be symptomatic depending on the degree and direction of radial head dislocation. Incomplete dislocations often produce early symptoms of pain and limited motion. In contrast, complete anterior dislocations may be asymptomatic or block terminal elbow flexion. Other findings at presentation are valgus elbow deformity and lateral prominence about the radial head. On occasion, the patient presents with neurologic symptoms, such as a posterior interosseous nerve palsy resulting from an anteriorly dislocated radial head or a tardy ulnar nerve palsy resulting from the valgus elbow deformity.[17] In the pediatric patient, prolonged dislocation causes the concave articular surface of the radial head to become convex and the capitellum to flatten.[17]

FIGURE 6

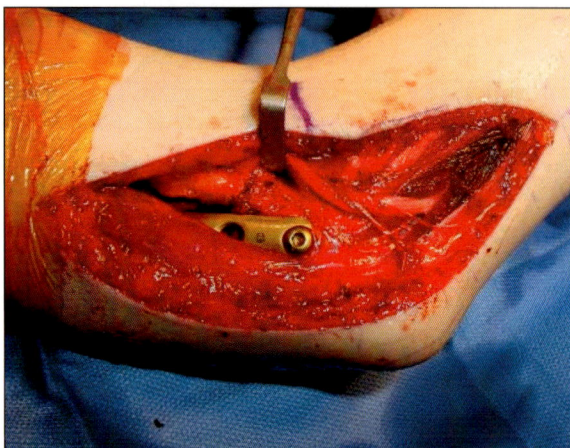

Clinical photograph shows supplemental medial incision to allow identification, retraction, and transposition of the ulnar nerve. In addition, the distal fragment can be translated in a medial direction to minimize lateral prominence. (Courtesy of Shriners Hospitals for Children, Philadelphia, PA.)

Commonly Used Childhood Interventions

The treatment of a missed Monteggia fracture-dislocation is controversial regarding the timing of treatment, the reducibility of chronic dislocations, opti-

FIGURE 7

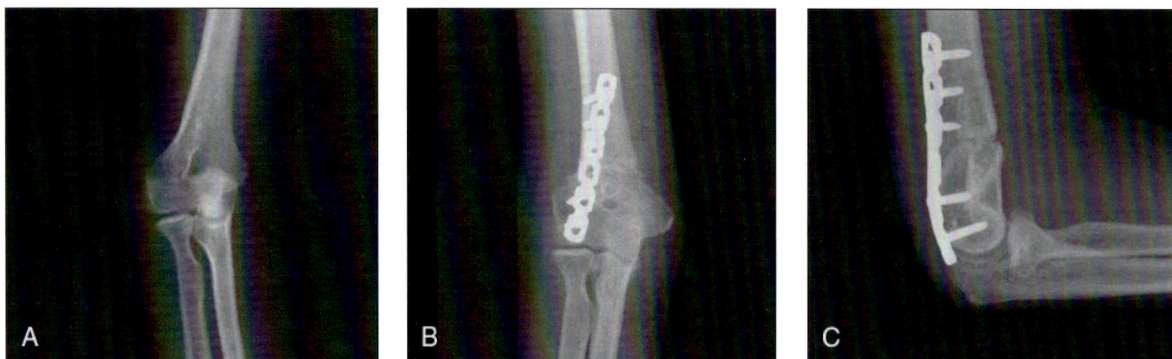

Radiographs of the right elbow of an 18-year-old woman with cubitus varus deformity treated with dome osteotomy. **A,** Preoperative AP view shows cubitus varus. **B,** Postoperative AP view shows dome osteotomy and internal fixation. **C,** Postoperative lateral view demonstrates posterolateral plate-and-screw configuration. (Courtesy of Shriners Hospitals for Children, Philadelphia, PA.)

FIGURE 8

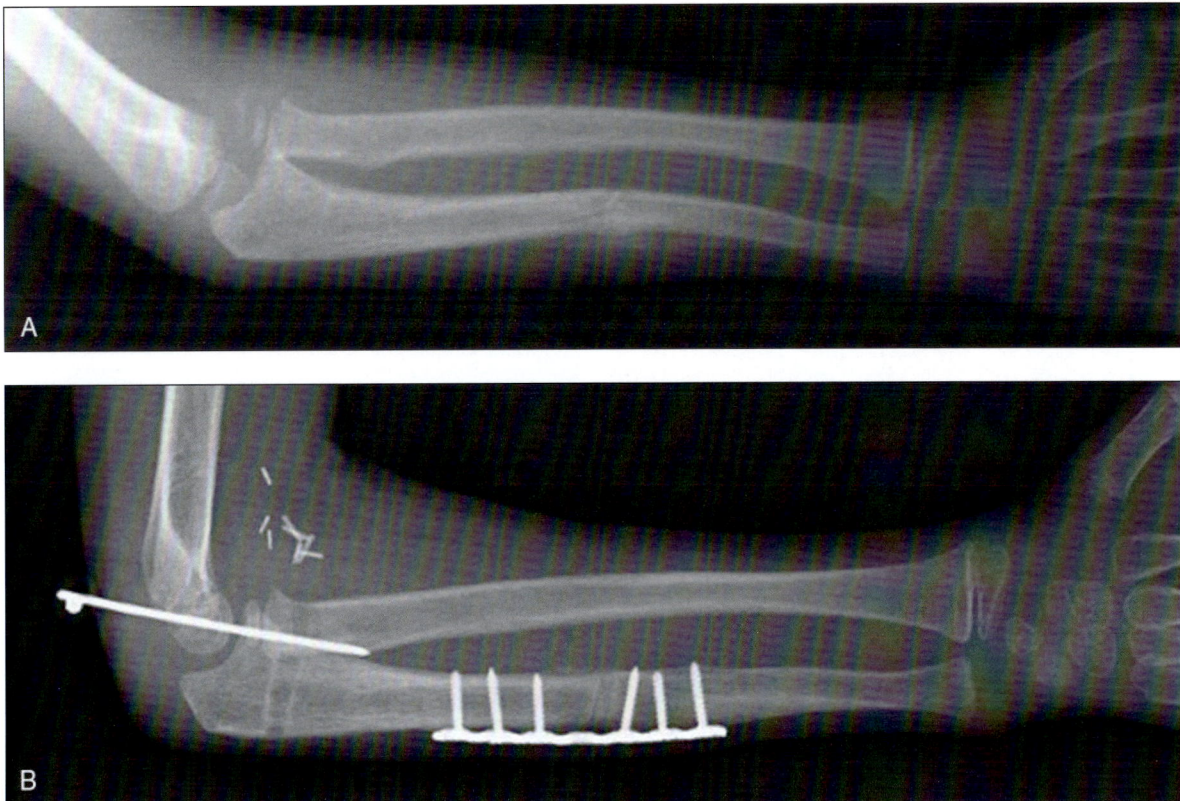

PA radiographs of the arm of a 10-year-old boy with a missed Monteggia fracture-dislocation and who underwent open reduction with corrective osteotomy of the ulna and annular ligament reconstruction. **A,** Preoperative view shows the radial head dislocated anteriorly and the ulna angulated anteriorly. **B,** Postoperative view. (Courtesy of Shriners Hospitals for Children, Philadelphia, PA.)

mum patient age, and the specific surgical technique.[18-22] Anecdotal reports suggest that successful surgical reduction can be accomplished up to 6 years postinjury in patients younger than 12 years. On the basis of objective measures, such as the Mayo Elbow Performance Index and radiographic follow-up evaluation, Nakamura et al[17] concluded that open reduction can be successfully performed in patients younger than 12 years or within 3 years of injury.

Interventions for the Adult Patient

Surgical options for the treatment of a Monteggia fracture-dislocation are similar in both adults and children and include reconstruction of the annular liga-ment,[23] corrective osteotomy of the ulna,[22] bending osteotomy of the ulna,[24] combined lengthening and bending osteotomy of the ulna,[18] gradual lengthening and angulation of the ulna,[25] osteotomy of the ulna combined with shortening of the radius,[19] and rotational osteotomy of the radius.[26] More recent reports support a combination of procedures to correct ulnar deformity and to reconstruct the annular ligament.[17,19-21] The mainstay of treatment is the correction of any ulnar deformity. Overcorrection of the ulnar deformity will facilitate radial head reduction. If the radial head fails to reduce, then open reduction and ligament reconstruction is necessary. In adults with markedly deformed and/or arthritic radial heads, simple excision may alleviate symptoms.

FIGURE 9

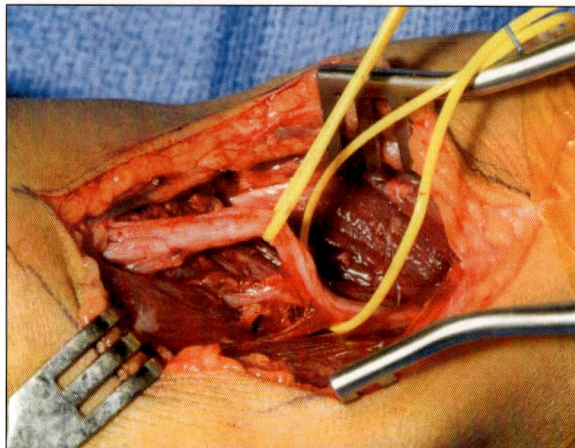

Clinical photograph shows identification and neurolysis of the radial nerve via an anterior Henry approach. (Courtesy of Shriners Hospitals for Children, Philadelphia, PA.)

FIGURE 10

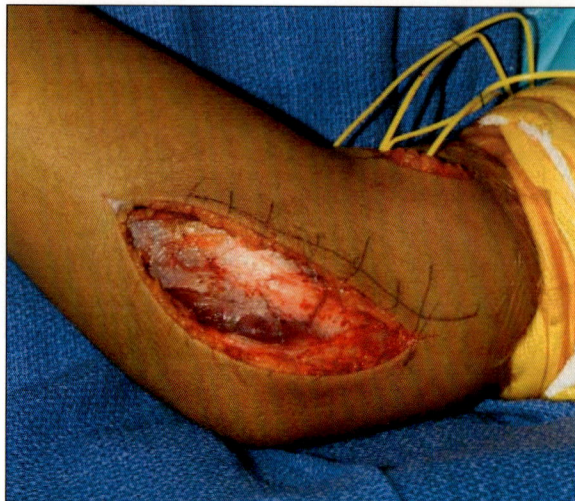

Clinical photograph shows the lateral Kocher approach to identify the ulnar malunion site and allow access to the radiocapitellar joint. (Courtesy of Shriners Hospitals for Children, Philadelphia, PA.)

Expert Opinion

Open reduction for a subacute or chronic Monteggia fracture-dislocation is difficult in both adults and children. The earlier the diagnosis is made, the easier the reduction will be. Most commonly, the radial head is dislocated anteriorly and the ulna is angulated or bowed in the same direction (**Figure 8, A**). First, the ulna must be corrected (and often, overcorrected) to allow radial head reduction (**Figure 8, B**). Second, the anteriorly dislocated radial head displaces the posterior interosseous nerve and the surgeon must either identify the nerve or be particularly aware of its position. In general, this chapter's authors prefer to identify the nerve via a separate anterior approach and decompress the nerve beneath the supinator. The separate approach also facilitates annular ligament reconstruction. Third, the surgeon must decide whether repair of the annular ligament remnant is sufficient to maintain the reduction or if reconstruction is necessary. When in doubt, reconstruction is preferred because the integrity of the annular ligament remnant is difficult to gauge.

An anterior Henry approach is performed and the radial nerve is identified between the brachialis and brachioradialis muscles (**Figure 9**). The sensory and posterior interosseous branches of the radial nerve are isolated and traced in a distal direction. The crossing vessels along the posterior interosseous nerve are ligated. The leading edge of the supinator muscle, or arcade of Fröhse, is released and the nerve is traced into the muscle. A separate lateral Kocher approach is performed, which is extended along the ulna to identify the malunion site (**Figure 10**). An ulnar osteotomy is performed and the bone is overcorrected and lengthened approximately 1 cm. Temporary fixation is accomplished using a bridge plate or an external fixator. A lateral arthrotomy is performed and the annular ligament is incised. All scar tissue within the radiocapitellar joint must be removed to allow concentric reduction (**Figure 11**). The radial head is reduced and aligned with the capitellum (**Figure 12**). Failure to attain reduction requires reassessment of the ulna and ensuring that all fibrous tissue has been removed from the joint.

After the radiocapitellar joint is reduced, the surgeon must either repair or reconstruct the annular ligament. Subacute cases are amenable to repair using nonabsorbable suture. Chronic cases require ligament reconstruction. The authors of this chapter prefer using a tendon graft, usually obtained from the flexor carpi radialis, to reconstruct the annular ligament. The authors use the Seel and Peterson[27] anatomic technique rather than the

FIGURE 11

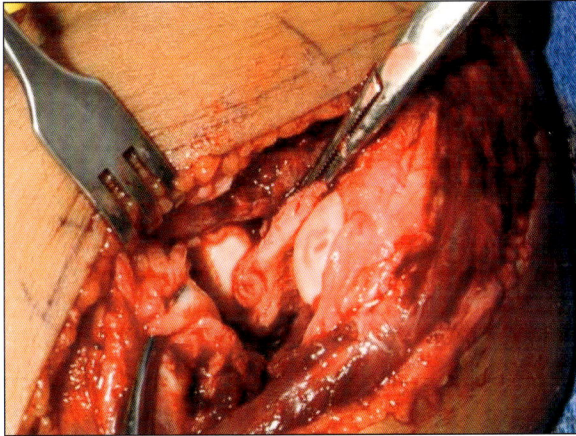

Clinical photograph shows lateral arthrotomy and all scar tissue removed from within the radiocapitellar joint. (Courtesy of Shriners Hospitals for Children, Philadelphia, PA.)

FIGURE 12

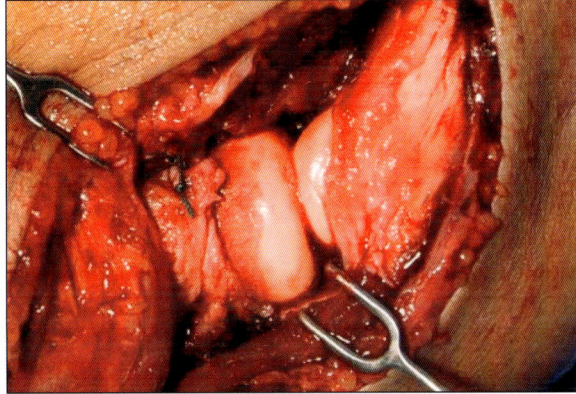

Clinical photograph shows the radial head reduced and aligned with the capitellum. (Courtesy of Shriners Hospitals for Children, Philadelphia, PA.)

Bell Tawse reconstruction.[28] Holes are drilled through the ulna about the proximal radioulnar joint using the anterior and posterior incisions. The radial head is reduced and the free tendon graft is placed around the radial neck and through the osseous tunnels (**Figure 8, B**). The graft is secured within the tunnel using interference screws or a docking technique. Supplemental K-wire fixation is controversial; if used, the wire is inserted from the posterior elbow across the capitellum and into the radial head.

LATERAL CONDYLE FRACTURES
Commonly Used Childhood Interventions
Lateral condylar fractures account for one fifth of distal humerus fractures in children.[29] Lateral condyle fracture is thought to occur as a result of forced varus angulation with the elbow extended and the forearm supinated.[30] Rutherford[31] reviewed 36 children with 39 fractures and noted 10 patients with malunion and only 1 patient with physeal arrest. Fracture nonunion and fishtail deformity of the distal humerus are sequelae that may present in the adult[31] (**Figure 13**). Fishtail deformity of the distal humerus is the result of osteonecrosis of the distal humeral epiphysis[32,33] and may also be noted in patients with lateral condyle fractures as well as other elbow fractures sustained in childhood. The natural

FIGURE 13

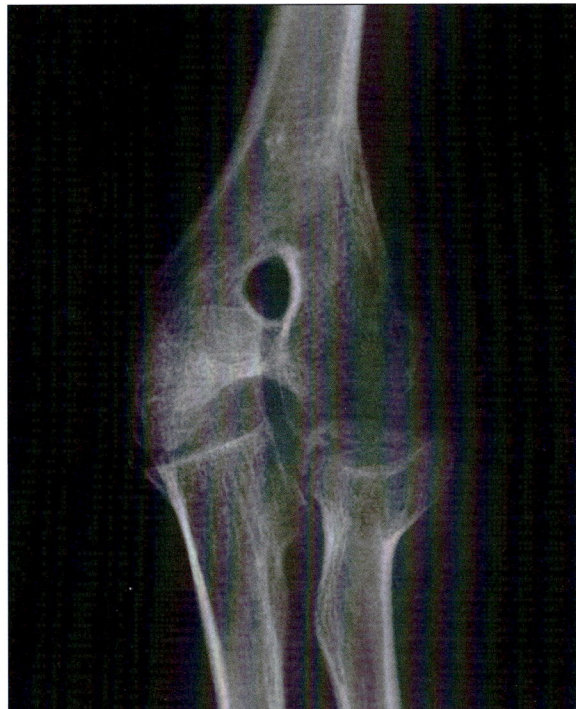

AP radiograph of a fishtail deformity of the distal humerus following a lateral condylar fracture. (Courtesy of Shriners Hospitals for Children, Philadelphia, PA.)

FIGURE 14

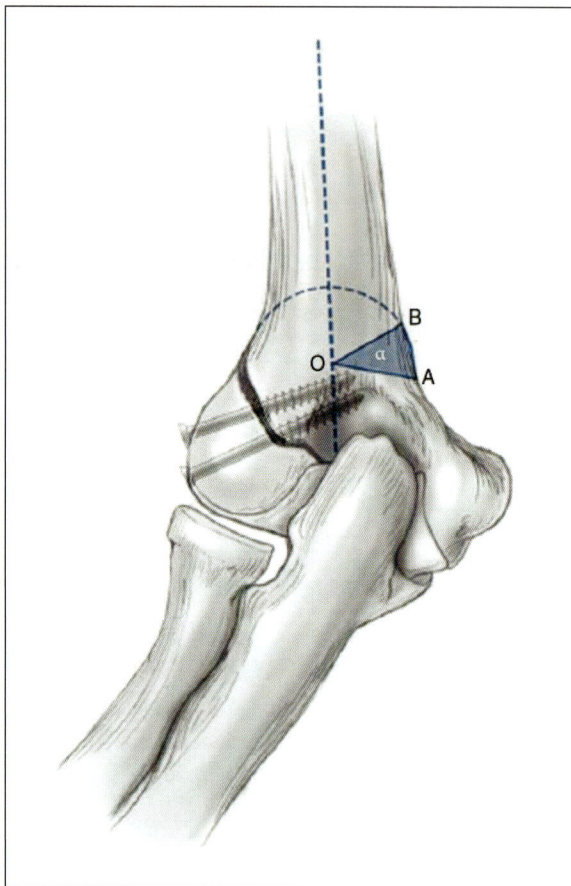

Illustration of a dome osteotomy. Point *A* is the junction between the periosteum and the perichondrium at the medial border of the distal humeral metaphysis. The intersection of the midline axis of the humerus and the proximal margin of the olecranon fossa (*O*) is designated at the center of the dome. With the *OA* segment as the base, a second line is drawn from point *O* to form an angle equal to the planned correction angle (α). Point *B* is the intersection of this line and the medial cortex. The length of segment *OB* is the radius of the dome. The arc of the dome osteotomy is defined on the basis of these parameters and is drawn with a methylene blue marking pen. (Reproduced with permission from Tien YC, Chen JC, Fu YC, Chih TT, Huang PJ, Wang GJ: Supracondylar dome osteotomy for cubitus valgus deformity associated with a lateral condylar nonunion in children: Surgical technique. *J Bone Joint Surg Am* 2006;88[Suppl 1 Pt 2]:191-201.)

history of a fishtail deformity varies.[34] Adolescents and adults may remain asymptomatic or develop intra-articular loose bodies and joint locking. In severe cases, progressive arthritis may develop, requiring interposition arthroplasty.

Outcomes

Lateral condylar nonunion with progressive valgus deformity of the elbow is a more common complication. This deformity can present in patients of all ages. The patient may present with pain, apprehension with use, deformity, or ulnar nerve symptoms. The goal of treatment is to achieve fracture union and to improve limb alignment. Lateral condylar nonunion without valgus deformity can be treated with in situ fixation. Lateral condylar nonunion with valgus deformity requires fixation and cubitus valgus correction. Extensive dissection of the lateral condyle can result in osteonecrosis, frank joint arthrosis, and degeneration of the elbow joint.[30,35-38]

Interventions for the Adult Patient

Tien et al[36] have described supracondylar dome osteotomy as an alternative treatment option that decreases the complication rate. A posterior midline incision is used at the distal humerus to visualize the nonunion site by mobilizing and retracting the triceps medially. The fibrous tissue at the nonunion site is excised and the fracture is reduced and fixed in situ with two cancellous compression screws but without bone graft. This technique avoids excessive soft-tissue dissection of the nonunion fragment and spares the physeal and epiphyseal surfaces.[36]

Following lateral condylar fixation, the proximal periosteum is incised in preparation for a dome osteotomy (**Figure 14**). The ulnar nerve is routinely transposed to relieve tension on the nerve. Postoperatively, elbow immobilization varies with the internal fixation technique. Rigid fixation allows early movement, whereas K-wires require 3 to 4 weeks of immobilization.[36]

Tien et al[37] reported on eight consecutive patients treated over a 6-year period. The mean interval between sustaining the lateral condylar fracture and undergoing surgery was 4.9 years. All eight lateral condylar nonunions achieved union within 3 months. All dome osteotomies healed uneventfully. The mean postoperative humerus-ulna angle was 5.5° of valgus. Overall results were graded as excellent in two patients, good in four patients, and fair in two patients.

FIGURE 15

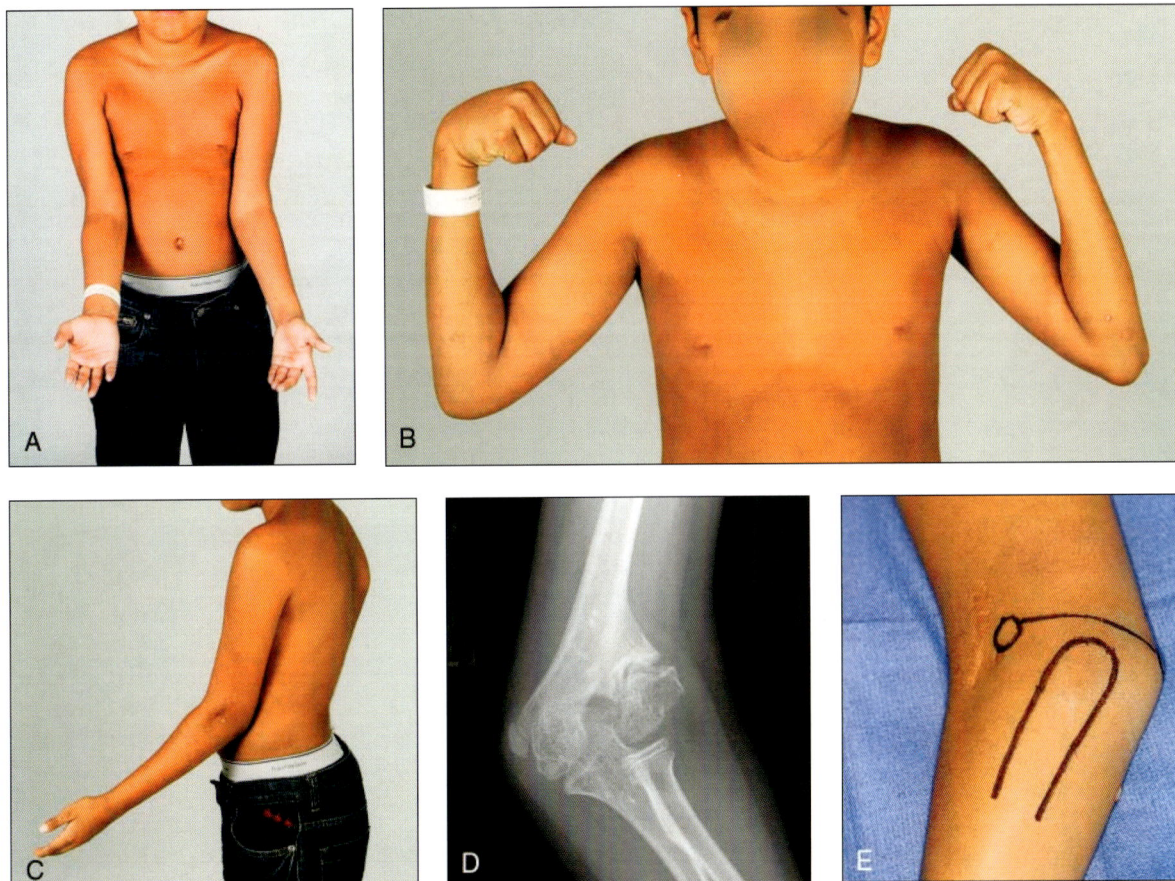

Images of a 10-year-old boy with lateral condylar nonunion in the left elbow who underwent dome osteotomy with internal fixation. Preoperative clinical photographs demonstrate left elbow cubitus valgus deformity (**A**), full flexion (**B**), and contracture (**C**). **D**, Preoperative AP radiograph shows lateral condylar nonunion. **E**, Photograph of the arm while the child is prone on the operating table with anatomic landmarks drawn on the posterior elbow. (continued)

Expert Opinion

Nonunion of a lateral condylar fracture is uncommon. Previously, the authors of this chapter used a two-stage approach to treatment: the first goal was to achieve lateral condylar union and the second was valgus malalignment correction. However, the authors considered the favorable results published by Tien et al[36,37] to be impressive. Based on the findings of Tien et al, the authors of this chapter now use a single-stage approach (**Figure 15**) following the principles outlined earlier and strive to achieve rigid fixation to allow earlier mobilization.

CONCLUSION

Most adult sequelae of pediatric conditions in the upper extremity relate to elbow fractures; specifically, supracondylar fractures of the distal humerus, Monteggia fracture-dislocations, and lateral condyle fractures. Recognition and appropriate treatment during childhood can prevent the development of these sequelae. Obtaining and maintaining appropriate alignment following these injuries is of the utmost importance.

FIGURE 15 (*continued*)

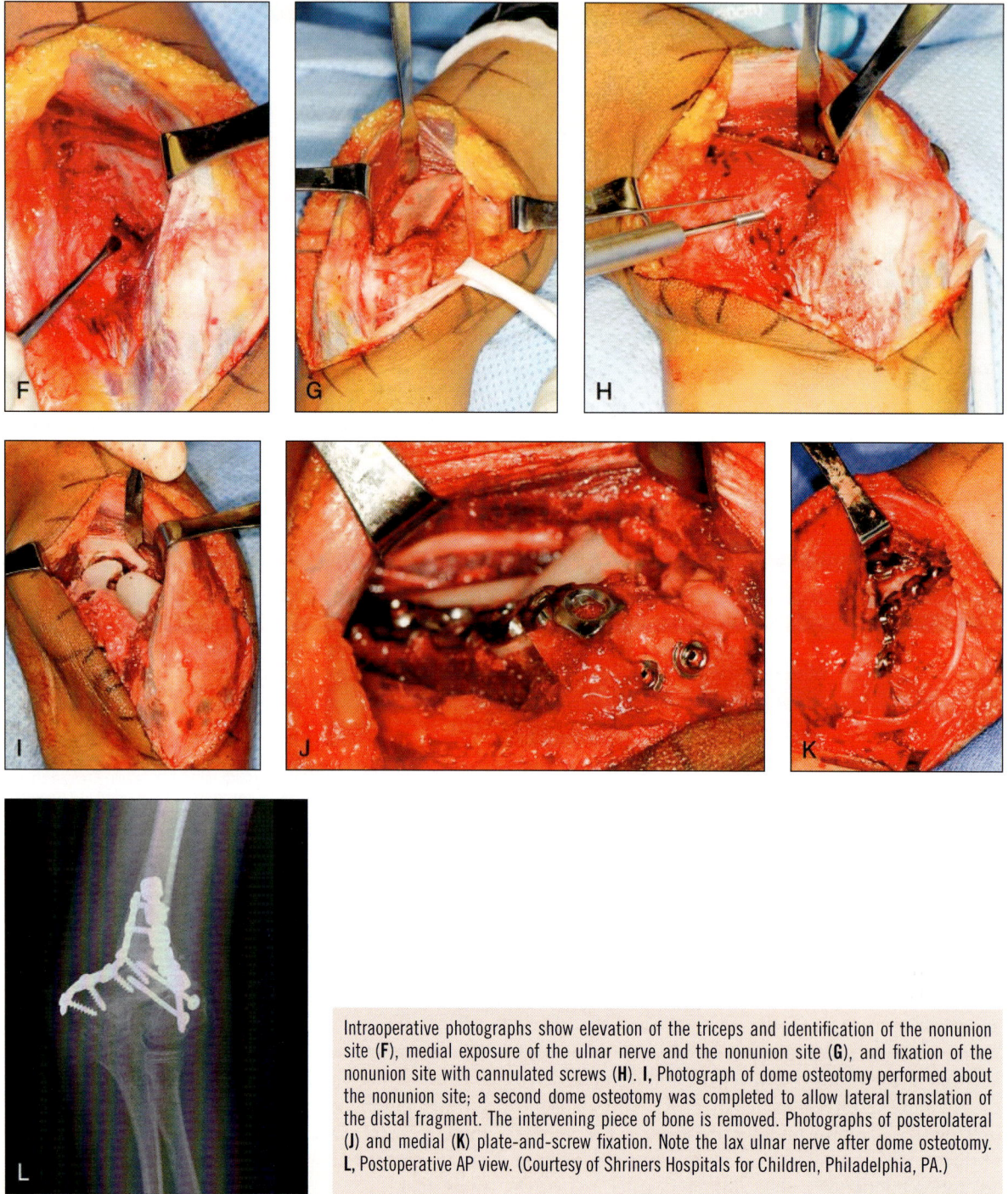

Intraoperative photographs show elevation of the triceps and identification of the nonunion site (**F**), medial exposure of the ulnar nerve and the nonunion site (**G**), and fixation of the nonunion site with cannulated screws (**H**). **I,** Photograph of dome osteotomy performed about the nonunion site; a second dome osteotomy was completed to allow lateral translation of the distal fragment. The intervening piece of bone is removed. Photographs of posterolateral (**J**) and medial (**K**) plate-and-screw fixation. Note the lax ulnar nerve after dome osteotomy. **L,** Postoperative AP view. (Courtesy of Shriners Hospitals for Children, Philadelphia, PA.)

REFERENCES

1. Otsuka NY, Kasser JR: Supracondylar fractures of the humerus in children. *J Am Acad Orthop Surg* 1997;5(1):19-26.

2. Dimeglio A: Growth in pediatric orthopaedics, in Morrissy RT, Weinstein SL, eds: *Lovell and Winter's Pediatric Orthopaedics*, ed 6. Philadelphia, PA., Lippincott Williams & Wilkins, 2005, vol 2, pp 35-65.

3. Cheng JC, Ng BK, Ying SY, Lam PK: A 10-year study of the changes in the pattern and treatment of 6,493 fractures. *J Pediatr Orthop* 1999;19(3):344-350.

4. Palmer EE, Niemann KM, Vesely D, Armstrong JH: Supracondylar fracture of the humerus in children. *J Bone Joint Surg Am* 1978;60(5):653-656.

5. Høyer A: Treatment of supracondylar fracture of the humerus by skeletal traction in an abduction splint. *J Bone Joint Surg Am* 1952;24-A(3):623-637.

6. Omid R, Choi PD, Skaggs DL: Supracondylar humeral fractures in children. *J Bone Joint Surg Am* 2008;90(5):1121-1132.

7. Takahara M, Sasaki I, Kimura T, Kato H, Minami A, Ogino T: Second fracture of the distal humerus after varus malunion of a supracondylar fracture in children. *J Bone Joint Surg Br* 1998;80(5):791-797.

8. Spinner RJ, O'Driscoll SW, Davids JR, Goldner RD: Cubitus varus associated with dislocation of both the medial portion of the triceps and the ulnar nerve. *J Hand Surg Am* 1999;24(4):718-726.

9. Abe M, Ishizu T, Nagaoka T, Onomura T: Recurrent posterior dislocation of the head of the radius in post-traumatic cubitus varus. *J Bone Joint Surg Br* 1995;77(4):582-585.

10. O'Driscoll SW, Spinner RJ, McKee MD, et al: Tardy posterolateral rotatory instability of the elbow due to cubitus varus. *J Bone Joint Surg Am* 2001;83-A(9): 1358-1369.

11. Beuerlein MJ, Reid JT, Schemitsch EH, McKee MD: Effect of distal humeral varus deformity on strain in the lateral ulnar collateral ligament and ulnohumeral joint stability. *J Bone Joint Surg Am* 2004;86-A(10):2235-2242.

12. Kumar K, Sharma VK, Sharma R, Maffulli N: Correction of cubitus varus by French or dome osteotomy: A comparative study. *J Trauma* 2000;49(4):717-721.

13. Pankaj A, Dua A, Malhotra R, Bhan S: Dome osteotomy for posttraumatic cubitus varus: A surgical technique

to avoid lateral condylar prominence. *J Pediatr Orthop* 2006;26(1):61-66.

14. French PR: Varus deformity of the elbow following supacondylar fractures of the humerus in children. *Lancet* 1959;2(7100):439-441.

15. Bellemore MC, Barrett IR, Middleton RW, Scougall JS, Whiteway DW: Supracondylar osteotomy of the humerus for correction of cubitus varus. *J Bone Joint Surg Br* 1984;66(4):566-572.

16. Kim HT, Lee JS, Yoo CI: Management of cubitus varus and valgus. *J Bone Joint Surg Am* 2005;87(4):771-780.

17. Nakamura K, Hirachi K, Uchiyama S, et al: Long-term clinical and radiographic outcomes after open reduction for missed Monteggia fracture-dislocations in children. *J Bone Joint Surg Am* 2009;91(6):1394-1404.

18. Hirayama T, Takemitsu Y, Yagihara K, Mikita A: Operation for chronic dislocation of the radial head in children: Reduction by osteotomy of the ulna. *J Bone Joint Surg Br* 1987;69(4):639-642.

19. Stoll TM, Willis RB, Paterson DC: Treatment of the missed Monteggia fracture in the child. *J Bone Joint Surg Br* 1992;74(3):436-440.

20. Horii E, Nakamura R, Koh S, Inagaki H, Yajima H, Nakao E: Surgical treatment for chronic radial head dislocation. *J Bone Joint Surg Am* 2002;84-A(7):1183-1188.

21. Wang MN, Chang WN: Chronic posttraumatic anterior dislocation of the radial head in children: Thirteen cases treated by open reduction, ulnar osteotomy, and annular ligament reconstruction through a Boyd incision. *J Orthop Trauma* 2006;20(1):1-5.

22. Best TN: Management of old unreduced Monteggia fracture dislocations of the elbow in children. *J Pediatr Orthop* 1994;14(2):193-199.

23. Hurst LC, Dubrow EN: Surgical treatment of symptomatic chronic radial head dislocation: A neglected Monteggia fracture. *J Pediatr Orthop* 1983;3(2):227-230.

24. Tajima T, Yoshizu T: Treatment of long-standing dislocation of the radial head in neglected Monteggia fractures. *J Hand Surg Am* 1995;20(3 Pt 2):S91-S94.

25. Exner GU: Missed chronic anterior Monteggia lesion: Closed reduction by gradual lengthening and angulation of the ulna. *J Bone Joint Surg Br* 2001;83(4):547-550.

26. Futami T, Tsukamoto Y, Fujita T: Rotation osteotomy for dislocation of the radial head: 6 cases followed for 7 (3-10) years. *Acta Orthop Scand* 1992;63(4):455-456.

27. Seel MJ, Peterson HA: Management of chronic post-traumatic radial head dislocation in children. *J Pediatr Orthop* 1999;19(3):306-312.

28. Bell Tawse AJ: The treatment of malunited anterior Monteggia fractures in children. *J Bone Joint Surg Br* 1965;47(4):718-723.

29. Blount WP: Fractures of the lateral condyle of the humerus, in *Fractures in Children*. Baltimore, MD, Williams and Wilkins, 1954, pp 43-45.

30. Jakob R, Fowles JV, Rang M, Kassab MT: Observations concerning fractures of the lateral humeral condyle in children. *J Bone Joint Surg Br* 1975;57(4):430-436.

31. Rutherford A: Fractures of the lateral humeral condyle in children. *J Bone Joint Surg Am* 1985;67(6):851-856.

32. McDonnell DP, Wilson JC: Fractures of the lower end of the humerus in children. *J Bone Joint Surg Am* 1948;30-A(2):347-358.

33. Wilson JN: Fractures of the external condyle of the humerus in children. *Br J Surg* 1955;43(177):88-94.

34. Morrissy RT, Wilkins KE: Deformity following distal humeral fracture in childhood. *J Bone Joint Surg Am* 1984;66(4):557-562.

35. Hardacre JA, Nahigian SH, Froimson AI, Brown JE: Fractures of the lateral condyle of the humerus in children. *J Bone Joint Surg Am* 1971;53(6):1083-1095.

36. Tien YC, Chen JC, Fu YC, Chih TT, Huang PJ, Wang GJ: Supracondylar dome osteotomy for cubitus valgus deformity associated with a lateral condylar nonunion in children: Surgical technique. *J Bone Joint Surg Am* 2006;88(Suppl 1 Pt 2):191-201.

37. Tien YC, Chen JC, Fu YC, Chih TT, Hunag PJ, Wang GJ: Supracondylar dome osteotomy for cubitus valgus deformity associated with a lateral condylar nonunion in children. *J Bone Joint Surg Am* 2005;87(7):1456-1463.

38. Shimada K, Masada K, Tada K, Yamamoto T: Osteosynthesis for the treatment of non-union of the lateral humeral condyle in children. *J Bone Joint Surg Am* 1997;79(2):234-240.

CHAPTER 8

LIMB-LENGTH DISCREPANCY AND BLOUNT DISEASE

JAMES J. MCCARTHY, MD

MATTHEW W. SQUIRE, MD, MS

MARTIN J. HERMAN, MD

LIMB-LENGTH DISCREPANCY

Limb-length discrepancy (LLD) is common in adults. Depending on the definition, more than one half of the US adult population may have a measurable LLD.[1] Twenty-three percent of adults have an LLD 1 cm or greater,[2] and 1 adult in 1,000 has an LLD greater than 2 cm, requiring use of a corrective device such as a shoe lift.[3] LLD is broadly classified in two different ways, and is commonly described either by its etiology or by the magnitude of the discrepancy.

LLDs generally are divided into one of two categories: congenital or acquired. A congenital LLD results from a congenital or genetic condition that alters the growth of the extremities. Limb hypoplasia syndromes, the most common of which is longitudinal deficiency of the fibula; hemihypertrophy syndromes, such as Klippel-Trenaunay-Weber syndrome; and global skeletal dysplasias are examples of congenital LLDs.

An acquired LLD results from an injury or disease process that affects a limb that was normal at birth. Fractures and bone infections that involve the physis of the femur or tibia, both of which may cause bony bar formation or damage to physeal cartilage growth, are the most common causes of acquired LLD in children. Pediatric hip diseases, such as developmental dysplasia of the hip (DDH), slipped capital femoral epiphysis (SCFE), and Legg-Calvé-Perthes disease, are common pediatric conditions that may result in a significant LLD because of either the conditions themselves or complications from their treatment. Neuromuscular diseases such as cerebral palsy also can cause differential limb growth over time. The etiology of the discrepancy is important to establish whenever possible. Some patients may actually benefit from a small LLD, such as children with hemiplegic cerebral palsy, poliomyelitis, or other neuromuscular disorders, because the shortening of the limb on the weak side, for example, may aid the patient in clearance during the swing phase of gait.[4]

LLDs are also classified by the magnitude of the inequality. In skeletally immature patients, the magnitude of the LLD guides treatment (**Table 1**). In any discussion of LLD, the magnitude of the deformity is based on radiographic assessment of the lower limbs, taking into account joint range of motion and clinical deformities of the pelvis and feet.

Commonly Used Childhood Interventions
Nonsurgical Treatment
For small LLDs, limb-length equalization can be accomplished with a shoe lift alone. The ideal shoe lift,

---

TABLE 1 General Guidelines for the Treatment of Limb-Length Inequality

LLD (cm)	Treatment
<2	Nonsurgical treatment (or using a shoe lift)
2–5	Epiphysiodesis or shortening procedure (if the patient is skeletally mature)
>5–15	Lengthening procedure
>15	Lengthening procedure (staged or combined with epiphysiodesis). Amputation, if lengthening procedure fails, at patient/parent request, or with other associated anomalies.

LLD = limb-length discrepancy.

regardless of type, should correct for approximately two thirds of the total inequality. A shoe lift as thick as 1 cm can be inserted in the shoe as an insole before discomfort arises from foot constriction against the upper part of the shoe or in the toebox. Larger discrepancies require the addition of rubber or other material to the sole of the shoe. This modification presents a problem for families and patients in some cases because all shoes that are routinely worn require modification and not all shoe styles can be easily adapted. An LLD that exceeds 5 cm is difficult to treat with a shoe lift. The modified shoe appears unsightly and patients often report instability about the foot and ankle with large lifts, especially on uneven surfaces. An ankle-foot orthosis can be used with large shoe lifts to increase stability. Another alternative for the management of a large LLD is a foot-in-foot prosthesis. This prosthesis is often used as a temporizing measure for very young children with a significant limb-length inequality and may cause a fixed equinus contracture of the ankle because the prosthesis is molded around a plantarflexed ankle to decrease the bulkiness of the prosthesis.

Surgical Treatment

Epiphysiodesis is a simple, reliable outpatient procedure with few complications.[5,6] One commonly used technique is percutaneous drilling. This fluoroscopically aided technique has resulted in physeal closure in 85% to 100% of patients, with few complications and good overall limb equalization.[7-10] Epiphysiodesis is performed on the long leg of the skeletally immature patient and requires the surgeon to make predictions about the degree of growth inhibition and the expected LLD at

maturity. Although epiphysiodesis is readily accepted by most patients and families, a few families think that operating on the unaffected leg and diminishing the patient's overall height is unappealing. Epiphysiodesis can also be used in combination with lengthening of the short leg in individuals with large inequalities who prefer to avoid a second or third lengthening procedure if the difference cannot be made up with a single lengthening procedure.

Shortening techniques are generally used after skeletal maturity to achieve leg length equality. Shortening is performed via an osteotomy of a predetermined length of bone that is then fixed with a blade plate or sideplate-and-screw construct (**Figure 1, A**) in the proximal femur or with intramedullary fixation in the diaphyseal femur (**Figure 1, B**) or tibia. Shortening is an accurate technique[11] and return to normal activity occurs in less time compared with lengthening techniques.[12]

Lengthening of the short limb can be performed in both children and adults, and is a time-consuming process that often requires months of active care and convalescence. Although many different techniques are used for limb lengthening, the most common is placement of an external frame that permits incremental bone lengthening via a diaphyseal or metaphyseal corticotomy site. In the typical patient, the limb is lengthened approximately 1 mm per day. After the desired length is achieved, the frame is then maintained for a prolonged period to allow bone consolidation. Because of extensive complication rates that can approach 100% in some cases, the surgeon should avoid lengthening of more than 20% of the bone's original length and carefully monitor patient progress.[13]

Outcomes

Children with limb-length inequalities that are left untreated do not commonly report pain and do not develop arthrosis to any significant degree. A large LLD that is left untreated results in a limp and increased energy expenditure when walking.[14] When standing in double-limb support with both knees extended, patients exhibit obligatory lumbar scoliosis that may become painful or result in a fixed deformity over time.

Children treated using the various methods of limb length equalization generally have improved gait and function.[15] Outcomes of treatment, however, are influenced by the etiology of the LLD, the degree of residual inequality remaining, and the effects of any complication that may have resulted from the treatment. For example, children with underlying congenital malformations, such as congenital femoral deficiency (that is, proximal femoral focal deficiency) treated using multiple lengthening procedures that often incorporate extensive hip and knee surgery, have worse overall outcomes than those who undergo a single lengthening procedure for posttraumatic growth arrest.

Adult Sequelae
Presenting Symptoms

Many musculoskeletal symptoms in adults, including gait deviation, back pain, scoliosis, and hip arthrosis, are attributed to LLD. Unfortunately, most studies regarding the long-term effects of LLDs in adults are retrospective case series and other studies with low levels of evidence. Limited literature on these topics makes drawing firm conclusions difficult regarding the connection between an existing LLD and the development of musculoskeletal problems in adults as they age.

Several authors have studied the functional effects of LLD on gait. Based on gait studies, significant gait asymmetry is seen only with an LLD of 2 cm or greater.[16] Inequalities less than 2 cm do not seem to alter the kinematics or kinetics of gait. Larger inequalities are associated with greater mechanical work during ambulation.[14] Equalization of limb length improves the symmetry of gait.[15]

The association between limb-length inequality and back pain in adults is controversial.[17-19] Because low back pain is very common in adults, attributing an LLD to the development and persistence of pain is difficult;

FIGURE 1

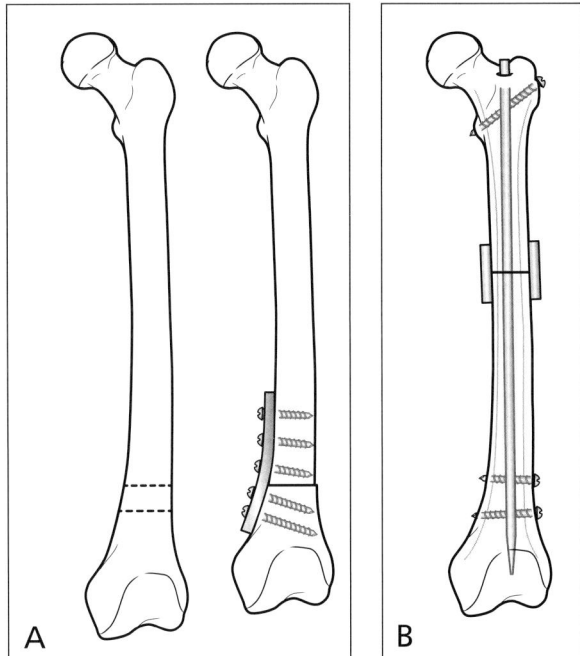

Illustrations show two limb shortening techniques. **A,** Sideplate-and-screw construct. **B,** Intramedullary fixation.

however, a small increase exists in the incidence of back pain in patients with LLDs. In one study of back pain in adults, only 8% of asymptomatic participants had an LLD greater than 1 cm, whereas almost 20% of patients with chronic back pain had an LLD greater than 1 cm.[20]

Other studies have been unable to link back pain with LLD.[17,18,21] Nourbakhsh and Arab[22] attempted to determine which patient factors were most closely associated with low back pain in adults. Poor endurance of the paraspinal extensor muscles was most highly correlated with symptomatic low back pain, whereas mechanical factors such LLD were not identified as important sources of pain. Several authors have evaluated the results of treatment of limb-length inequality, either with a shoe lift or with surgery, on low back pain.[23,24] For some patients, equalization of the LLD improves low back pain symptoms, whereas for others, it has no appreciable effect.

Some patients with a significant limb-length inequality who are examined in a standing position demonstrate clinical signs of scoliosis. The typical spinal deformity associated with an LLD is a lumbar curve with an apex that points to the long leg and is associated with a small degree of pelvic obliquity. Typically, curves secondary to an LLD are small and do not have severe apical rotation or significant secondary or double-curve patterns. Scoliosis that results primarily from an LLD typically is compensatory and flexible. Assessing the patient's spinal alignment in a sitting position or while standing after placing an appropriate-size shoe lift under the short leg is useful to distinguish a fixed deformity from one that compensates for the LLD. Supine bending radiographs of the spine also may be used to better assess the structural nature of spinal curves.

Some reports, however, have shown that not all curve patterns in patients with an LLD are the same.[25] In as many as one third of patients with a measureable lower limb discrepancy, the lumbar curve pattern is opposite to what is expected with an LLD.[21] In some adult patients with an LLD and scoliosis, radiographs confirm not only the scoliosis but any associated degenerative changes of the lumbar spine. This suggests that some scoliosis associated with an LLD in adults may be degenerative in nature and not strictly a result of pelvic obliquity.[20,26] In addition, some patients can have both an LLD and idiopathic scoliosis.

The effect of an LLD on the long lower limb is also controversial. One biomechanical model showed a 5% decrease in the weight-bearing contact surface of the hip of the long leg for every 1 cm of the LLD.[27] This decrease is partially explained by the fact that, in a double-leg stance with the weight equally distributed between both limbs, the hip of the long leg is positioned in slight adduction from the opposite limb. Brand and Yack[28] have concluded that the forces across the hip of the long leg are higher than the forces across the hip of the short leg. Friberg[26] observed that patients with an LLD who do not have a history of pediatric hip disease more commonly develop arthrosis in the hip of the longer leg compared with the short leg.

Physical Examination

Some adults can present primarily with an LLD that either has not been diagnosed previously or is the result of a traumatic injury in adulthood. Others may be experiencing problems related to a pediatric condition associated with an LLD. Some patients present primar-

ily with back or hip pain and are unaware of an LLD. A careful history should focus on the onset, location, and quality of the pain and identify any other signs or symptoms that are associated with it, such as sensory or motor changes in the legs or loss of joint mobility. Even when a patient has a known LLD, the orthopaedic surgeon must exclude other disease processes that may be the cause of the patient's symptoms before attributing them to the LLD. Additionally, the surgeon should inquire about the patient's medical history, occupation, leisure activities, and other lifestyle demands before making treatment decisions.

The patient is first observed walking so that the degree of gait disturbance may be identified. Overall muscle strength and coordination, joint mobility, and pain associated with weight bearing are assessed. The pelvis and lower limbs are inspected for malalignment or other deformities and soft-tissue abnormalities such as vascular malformations or skin lesions. Range of motion of the spine, hip, knee, and ankle is then determined. A pertinent neurologic examination completes the primary orthopaedic evaluation.

Leg length may be assessed in several ways. With the patient standing and with both knees and hips extended and in neutral abduction/adduction, the height of both iliac crests is determined by examining the patient from behind. Iliac crests that are obviously at different heights indicate an LLD. Blocks of known height can then be placed under the foot of the short limb, allowing the surgeon to estimate the magnitude of the discrepancy by recording the height of the block or blocks that most closely levels the iliac crests. Alternately, a tape measure can be used to determine the distance from the anterior superior iliac spine to the tip of the medial malleolus on both limbs. The Galeazzi test, typically used to assess hip dislocation in children, can also be used for clinical assessment of a patient with an LLD. With the patient supine and the hips and knees flexed, the height of the knees is determined. The knees will be different heights from the table in a patient with an LLD. The Galeazzi test is particularly useful for patients with hip or knee flexion contractures. Of the clinical methods for determining an LLD, leveling the pelvis with blocks placed under the short limb is the most accurate. Gross determination of the LLD using any of these methods, however, does not reveal the cause of the LLD. Although

FIGURE 2

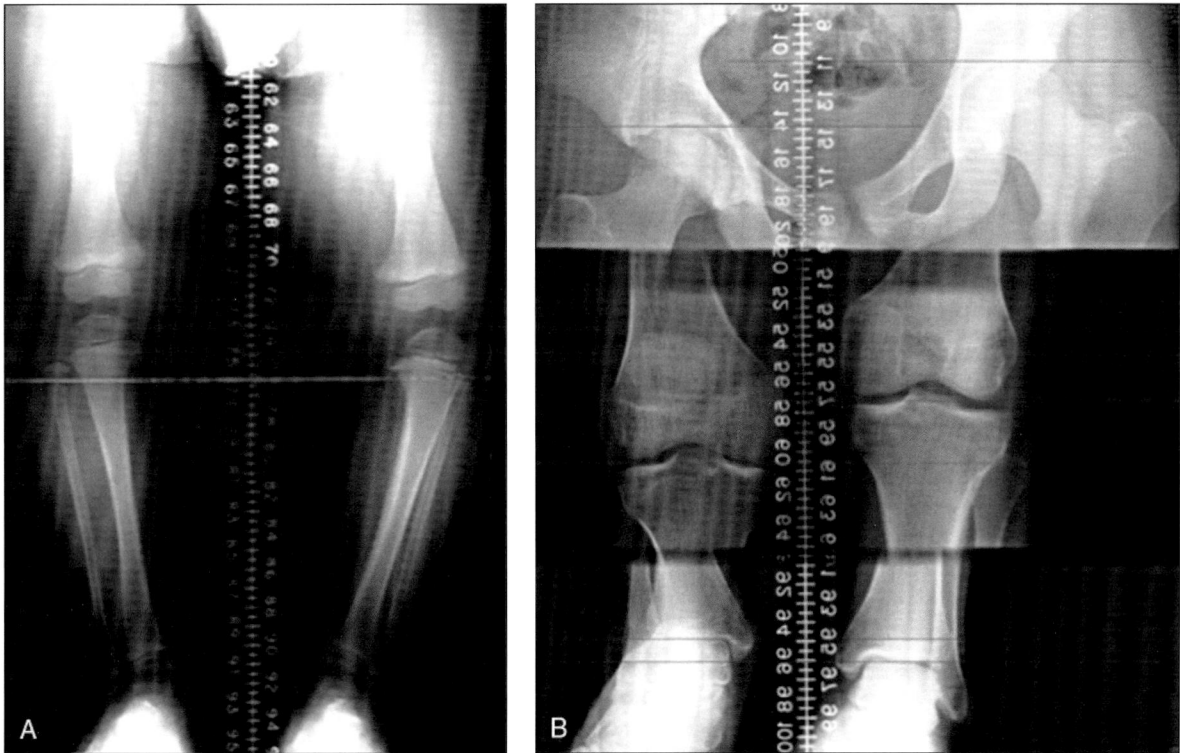

Imaging used to visualize and evaluate limb-length discrepancies (LLDs). **A,** Single-exposure AP radiograph (teleoradiograph) reveals the extent of the LLD. **B,** Scanograph shows three exposures (hip, knee, and ankle) on a single cassette to reduce measurement errors.

discrepancy of the lengths of the femora or tibias is most common, pelvic asymmetry, hip dislocation, joint contractures, and foot abnormalities are also potential causes of an LLD.

Imaging Studies

Various imaging techniques are routinely used to assess LLD. Radiographic methods are the most accurate way to precisely determine an LLD. The teleoradiograph is a single-exposure AP radiograph of the lower extremities obtained with a ruler placed along the limb to be measured (**Figure 2, A**). Although this method is subject to a magnification error of 5% to 10%, it allows the surgeon to not only assess the lengths of the femur and tibia but also reveals coronal (angular) limb deformities and is not subject to movement errors.[29] The orthoradiograph incorporates three separate exposures

(hip, knee, and ankle) in an effort to avoid magnification errors. Scanography uses a similar technique, but the exposure size is reduced and all three exposures are obtained on one film cassette (**Figure 2, B**). Direct measurement of the orthoradiograph has been shown to be more accurate than using a radiolucent ruler.[30] Both orthoradiography and scanography are subject to movement errors, and angular deformities cannot be assessed. All of these standard radiographic techniques are inaccurate if the patient has knee or hip flexion contractures, or if the lower extremities are held in different positions. Lateral radiographs or separate (prone) AP radiographs of the femur and tibia obtained while a ruler is placed next to the limb can be used to assess limb length in patients with knee flexion contractures.

CT has become increasingly popular for the assessment of limb length and has replaced other radiographic techniques in some centers.[31] Radiation exposure with CT is increased compared with scanography. CT is generally considered more accurate than conventional radiographic techniques, especially for patients with knee or hip flexion contractures[4] and complex limb deformities.

Errors can be made in determining an LLD using the various imaging techniques. Misplacement of the ruler, variations in the distance of the radiation source, and mathematic errors by the surgeon are some of the common pitfalls with radiographic techniques. CT measurements may be affected by the patient's positioning in the gantry; actual measurements are obtained by the technician or radiologist, preventing the surgeon from making his or her own determinations. All of these imaging methods are more prone to error when the patient has a complex deformity, contractures, or is unable to cooperate or stay motionless during imaging.

Interventions for the Adult Patient
Nonsurgical Treatment
Nonsurgical treatment consists primarily of a shoe lift; many of the same considerations that apply to the child also apply to the adult when prescribing a shoe lift. Most patients are most comfortable when approximately two thirds of the LLD is corrected and are comfortable with an in-shoe lift that measures up to 0.5 inch. Larger lifts must be incorporated into the sole of the shoe. Lifts larger than 5 cm often result in instability when the patient walks on uneven surfaces, increasing the risk of ankle injuries. Orthotic stabilization of the ankle in conjunction with the lift and prosthetics are options for adults with larger LLDs.

Surgical Treatment
In the adult, surgical intervention depends on the magnitude as well as the etiology of the discrepancy. LLD correction by shortening the longer limb or lengthening the shorter limb are both commonly used for adults with a significant LLD but without severe hip arthrosis. For those patients with an LLD and symptomatic degenerative joint disease (DJD) of the hip, limb-length equalization can also be accomplished at the time of total hip arthroplasty (THA).

Limb shortening is indicated in skeletally mature patients with an LLD of 2 to 6 cm[11,32,33] (**Figure 1**). Shortening is a reliable, accurate method of obtaining limb

equalization with few complications. Although closed intramedullary femoral shortening is the technique most commonly used for adults with a moderate LLD, other options such as subtrochanteric shortening with plate fixation, step-cut osteotomy, and shortening of the tibia have all been successfully used to equalize limb lengths.[34-37] Although more technically demanding than shortening alone, rotational and angular corrections can be incorporated into the shortening procedure.[38]

Compared with limb lengthening techniques, fewer complications can be expected after shortening and recovery from the procedure is generally faster. Quadriceps weakness is the complication that patients experience most often after shortening of the middiaphyseal femur, the most common site of shortening. To diminish the occurrence of this complication, most surgeons will not shorten the femur more than 10% of its length. Femoral shortening performed via a proximal osteotomy is an option that may cause less quadriceps weakness in some patients but requires more extensive surgical exposure.

Tibial shortening is performed less often than femoral shortening, and in a manner similar to femoral shortening via diaphyseal osteotomy fixed with an intramedullary nail. Tibial shortening greater than 3 to 4 cm results in a bulky appearance of the calf and weakness in plantar flexion. Additionally, serious complications such as nonunion and compartment syndrome of the lower leg may occur after tibial shortening.[35,38] Prophylactic compartment release is recommended at the time of tibial shortening.

Nonarthroplasty limb-lengthening procedures are routinely used to manage moderate to severe LLDs in adults. Techiques that require external frames are the most commonly used methods of lengthening; however, techniques are evolving that allow for more accurate correction, less time in the fixator, and more rapid consolidation of the newly formed bone. Several designs for completely implantable intramedullary devices are now being used. The advantages of intramedullary devices include immediate axial stability, prevention of angular deformity during bone lengthening, elimination of pin tract infections, and minimal scarring.[39] The use of growth factors such as bone morphogenetic protein, electric stimulation, and ultrasound to speed consolidation is another important advancement and an ever-

FIGURE 3

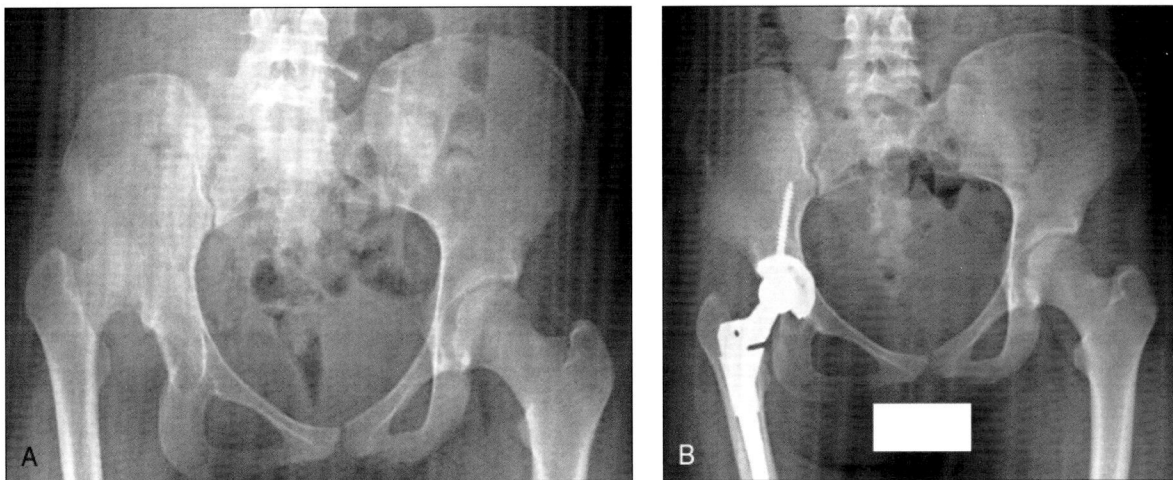

Supine AP radiographs of a 35-year-old patient with a history of developmental hip dysplasia who underwent total hip arthroplasty to correct a limb-length discrepancy (LLD). **A,** Preoperative view shows inequality at the right hip joint with an LLD of approximately 3 cm. **B,** Postoperative view shows hip joint equalization achieved by placing the cup at the level of the true acetabulum and LLD correction.

growing field of study.[40] Other techniques such as using transplanted cells (cultured stem cells or autologous chondrocyte cells) or altering the growth rate via systemic growth factors are potentially less invasive methods of limb-length equalization and angular correction.[41]

Adults who commit to limb lengthening must be counseled carefully about the pain and disability he or she will endure while undergoing the procedure, the potential for prolonged time missed from work or school, and the risks involved. Adult complications of limb lengthening, including infections related to the external frame, joint stiffness and subluxation, nerve injuries, and nonunion, as well as other problems must be disclosed frankly before proceeding with this complicated undertaking. For the surgeon, patient selection and preparation is perhaps the most important factor in achieving a good outcome.

THA is a common surgical technique that can be modified to improve LLD in adults who also have symptomatic hip arthritis (**Figure 3**). Lengthening or shortening can be accomplished by adjusting the length of the proximal femur during femoral component placement or by altering the hip center of rotation (acetabular component positioning). Significant limb lengthening at the time of THA is possible but

should be considered a secondary goal. In some cases, complete correction of the LLD at the time of THA may not be advisable or possible because of the magnitude of the preoperative discrepancy. The primary risk of limb lengthening performed in combination with THA is nerve injury, resulting from either excessive traction of the sciatic, femoral, or peroneal nerves or from direct nerve injury. Schmalzried et al[42] conducted a study of more than 3,000 patients who underwent THA and found that lengthening greater than 3 cm and procedures performed in patients with hip arthritis secondary to DDH were the most important risk factors for the development of nerve injuries. In another large study of patients who underwent THA for DDH, Eggli et al[43] showed that the risk of nerve palsy for patients who had undergone less than 3 cm of lengthening was the same as for those who had undergone 3 to 5 cm of lengthening. The authors concluded that the risk of nerve palsy correlated best with the technical complexity and time required to perform THA, not the magnitude of the lengthening.

Limb length equalization by shortening the long leg at the time of THA introduces other complications. Shortening more than 1 cm can result in significant postoperative abductor weakness and a Trendelenburg gait. This degree of shortening also can result in pros-thetic instability. Therefore, patients with a significantly longer leg on the side that will undergo THA should be counseled that their LLD may not be completely corrected. If significant shortening through the hip is planned, appropriate modifications of the surgical ap-proach that minimize dissection of the hip abductors and the use of a large articulation or a constrained ar-ticulation should be considered.

Expert Opinion
Patient Evaluation

Patient evaluation begins with a clinical examination, as described earlier in this chapter. The authors of this chapter prefer to assess the LLD using a weight-bearing long-leg AP radiograph that spans from the hip to the ankle. This radiograph is ideally obtained using a single long cassette from a focal distance of 10 ft. The authors of this chapter prefer this method because it allows eval-uation of limb deformity as well as the LLD. Additional imaging studies such as CT are obtained only for pa-tients with specific needs.

A trial of a shoe lift can be very helpful, not only to determine if the symptoms are related to the LLD but also to help the patient test-trial the limb correction. By varying the height of the lift applied, this trial also helps the clinicians, with the patient's input, to determine more accurately the exact degree of correction required.

Preferred Interventions

Because understanding of the adult sequelae of an LLD is limited, the decision to perform interventions, es-pecially surgical ones, must include a careful analysis of the risks and potential benefits. Patient education is critical so that the surgeon may match patient ex-pectations with possible outcomes. Judicious use of a shoe lift may be all that is required to improve gait and symptoms. Limb shortening and lengthening are also satisfactory options for patients with a significant LLD; improvements in gait and relief of pain generally can be expected. When an LLD occurs in conjunction with symptomatic hip arthrosis, THA modified to improve the LLD is a safe procedure when performed by experi-enced surgeons.

The surgical intervention must be carefully tailored to the patient, and the surgeon must be comfortable with a variety of limb correction techniques. No single tech-nique can be applied to all patients. Limb shortening will typically result in a quicker return to activities, of-ten allowing immediate weight bearing. For most work-ing adults, this represents the best option, especially if the discrepancy is in the femur. Nonarthroplasty length-ening techniques can be accomplished with external or intramedullary devices but all have high complication rates and require a lengthy convalescence. A thorough discussion with the patient and the family, over several office visits if necessary, about expected outcomes of the procedure and potential complications is best for both the patient and surgeon.

When hip arthrosis and an LLD coexist in the same limb, the discrepancy is grossly quantified in three dif-ferent ways: by asking the patient what size shoe lift he or she wears, by altering the limb lengths using wooden blocks until the patient feels his or her leg lengths have been equalized, and by radiographic measurements of magnification-adjusted pelvic radiographs. If a patient has a significant LLD and joint arthrosis, most LLDs can be improved at the time of THA. When a significant difference exists between a measured radiographic LLD and the patient-preferred block height that equalizes the leg lengths, we prefer to lengthen the limb to the amount preferred by the patient. Patients are counseled that risk of nerve palsy increases with lengthening procedures, and that, in some cases, significant limb lengthening cannot be achieved because of long-standing soft-tissue contractures. In the experience of this chapter's authors, lengthening is typically limited to 4 cm or less because of concerns regarding nerve palsy.

Blount Disease
Incidence of Pediatric Condition

Blount disease is the abnormal growth and development of the proximal medial tibia that results in varus angula-tion of the proximal tibia.[44] An increased posterior slope of the proximal medial tibia, sloping of the medial tibial plateau, internal rotation of the tibia, varus angulation of the distal femur (in late-onset forms), and LLD (in unilateral cases) are other manifestations of Blount dis-ease that influence treatment.

The prevalence of Blount disease is less than 1% in the general population and occurs typically in younger children (early or infantile) (**Figure 4**) or in adolescents

FIGURE 4

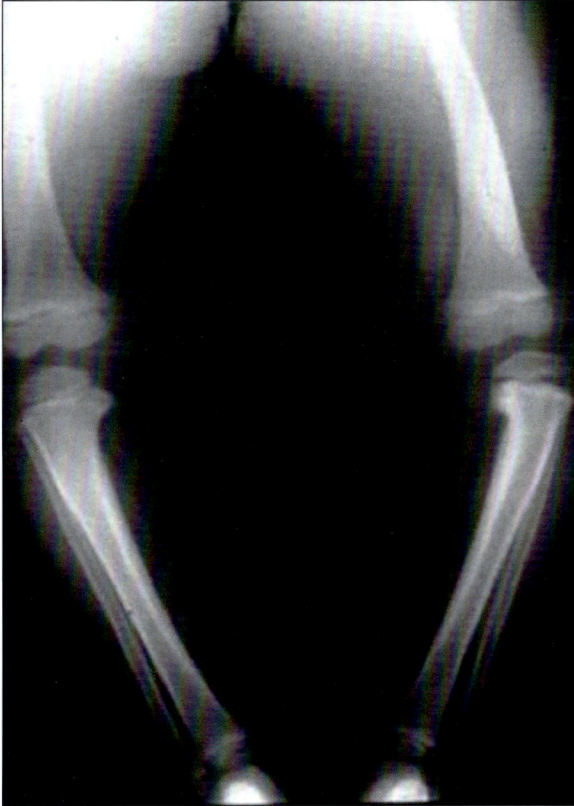

AP radiograph of infantile Blount disease in a 30-month-old child.

FIGURE 5

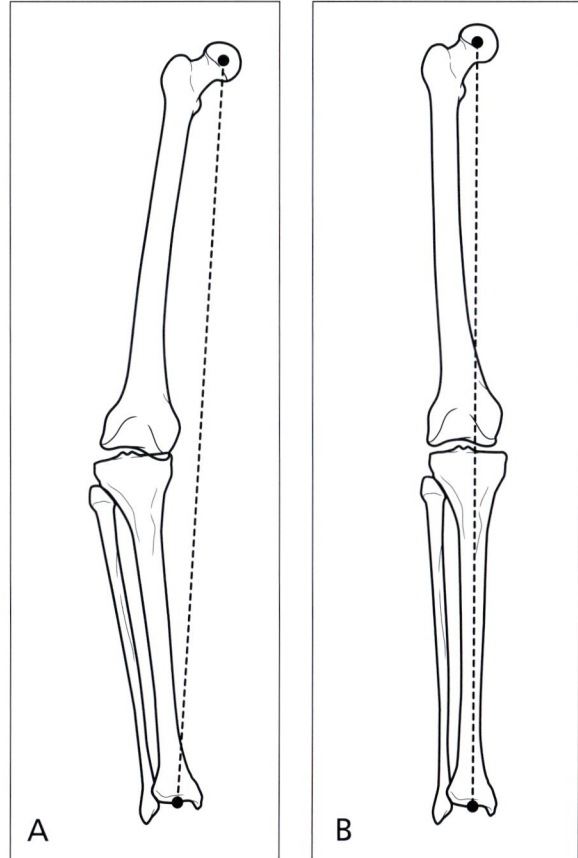

Illustrations show the goal of treating Blount disease in the lower limb. **A,** The mechanical axis (dashed line) is drawn from the center of the femoral head to the center of the ankle joint and lies just medial to the knee joint. A medial deviation of the axis indicates excessive forces distributed across the medial compartment of the knee and leads to the appearance of a bowed leg. **B,** Ideal correction of the disturbance restores the normal mechanical axis and allows a more even distribution of forces across the knee joint.

(late onset). In infants, the degree of deformity can vary widely from mild forms that are difficult to distinguish from physiologic bowing to severe forms that require surgical intervention and are associated with high recurrence rates even with optimal treatment. In older children and adolescents, the disease manifests most commonly in obese children, with knee pain and progressive genu varum. Rickets, metabolic bone diseases, and skeletal dysplasias are often associated with lower extremity bowing that must be distinguished from Blount disease.

Commonly Used Childhood Interventions
Nonsurgical Treatment
The goal of treatment is to restore the disturbed mechanical axis of the lower limb (**Figure 5**). Nonsurgical in-

terventions in children vary from simple observation to early bracing. Spontaneous resolution of mild cases of infantile Blount disease is common. Long leg bracing is the most common nonsurgical intervention for children older than 18 months with radiographic evidence of the earlier forms of the disease. The most commonly prescribed brace is a knee-ankle-foot orthosis. When used with the knee locked in extension, the knee-ankle-

FIGURE 6

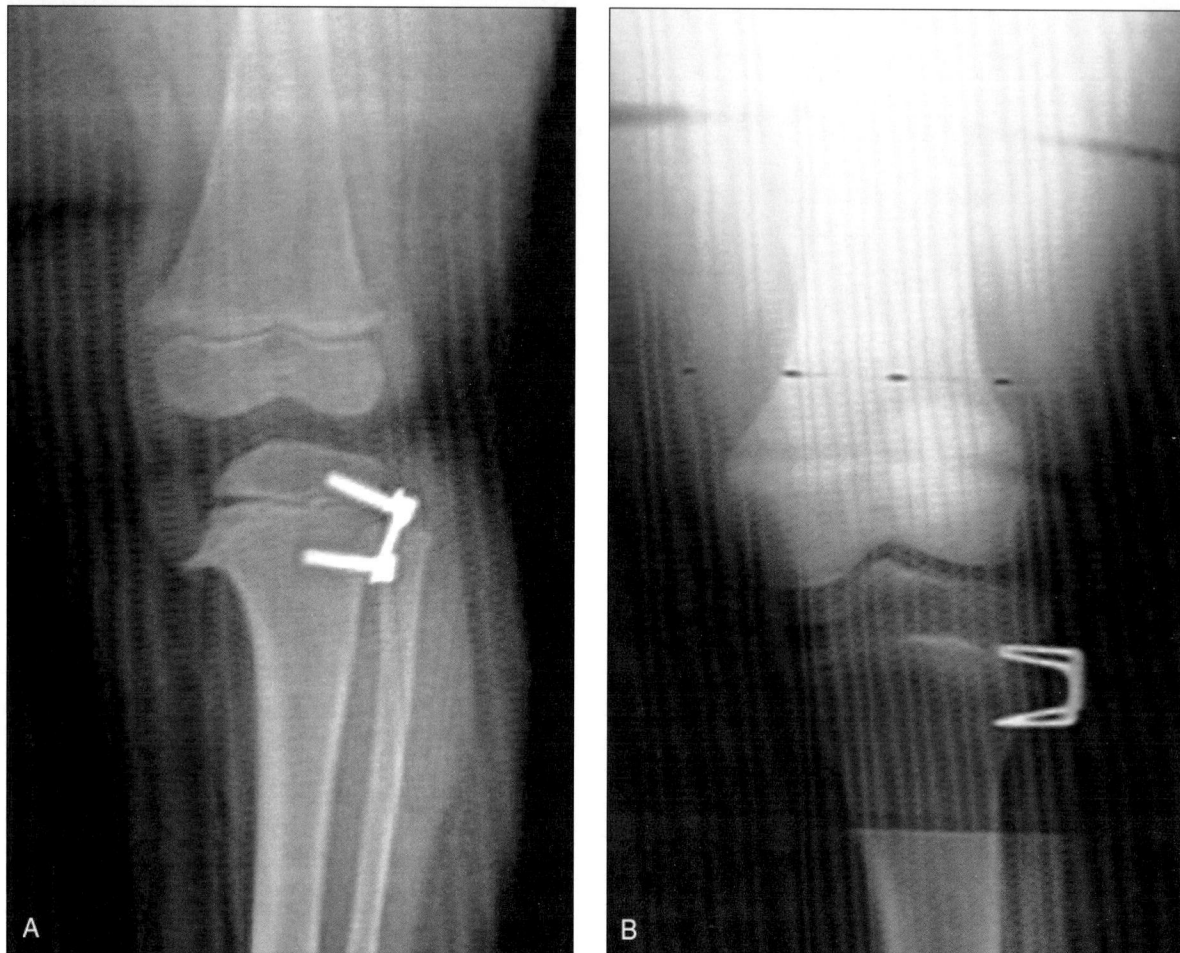

Postoperative weight-bearing AP radiographs demonstrate guided growth techniques used to correct the deformity angle in the knee secondary to Blount disease. **A,** View of the knee of a 4-year-old child with Blount disease obtained at 8-month follow-up. A plate-and-screw construct in the lateral proximal tibia inhibits lateral growth of the physis. Note the screws, which were placed parallel, are now splayed, indicating growth of the medial side. **B,** View of a knee obtained 2 years after placement of two lateral proximal tibial staples shows normal alignment.

foot orthosis is designed to apply a valgus force across the proximal tibia. Many infantile cases either resolve spontaneously or respond to brace treatment.[45] Bracing is not effective for adolescent Blount disease.

Surgical Treatment

Guided growth techniques are commonly used in the management of Blount disease by tethering the growth of the healthy lateral part of the proximal tibia to permit angular correction of the deformity with ongoing medial side growth (**Figure 6**). Guided growth techniques traditionally were limited to temporary spanning of the lateral proximal tibia with staples or surgical hemiepiphysiodesis and were used for mild to moderate disease in older children and adolescents. The more recent introduction of plate-screw constructs in place of staples has made guided growth a safe and reliable method of management for nonsevere Blount disease at any age.[46]

FIGURE 7

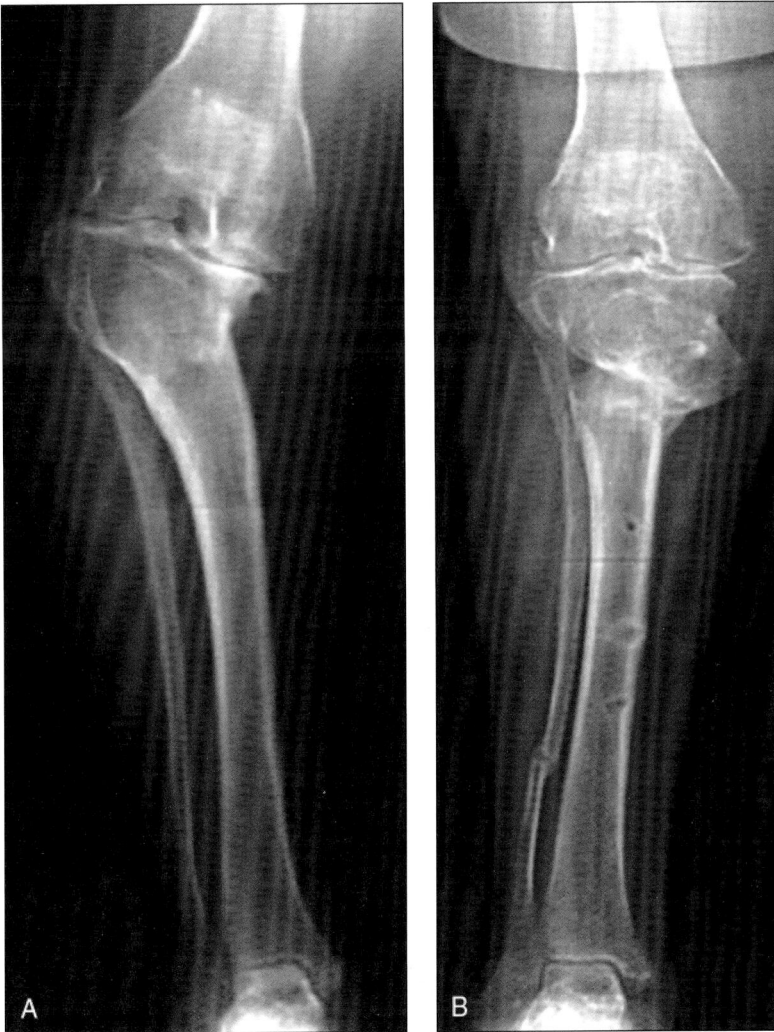

Weight-bearing AP radiographs of a severe lower limb deformity associated with Blount disease corrected using a tibial osteotomy and an external fixator. **A,** Preoperative view shows a bowed leg. **B,** Postoperative view shows the corrected deformity.

Tibial osteotomies are the mainstay of surgical intervention in children of all ages with severe Blount disease. For the infantile form, acute correction from varus to 10° of valgus held with internal fixation and casting is the mainstay of surgical treatment. For older children and adolescents, osteotomy and gradual correction with an external frame is the most common treatment (**Figure 7**). Although acute correction remains an option, complication rates historically have been higher compared with gradual correction techniques. The most serious complications are compartment syndrome and peroneal nerve palsy.[47-49]

Outcomes

The clinical course of untreated Blount disease is not well known. In addition to deformity, children and adolescents with Blount disease sometimes experience knee pain, especially with prolonged walking. This pain is likely the result of abnormal contact forces on the hyaline cartilage and menisci in the knee or lateral knee instability resulting from varus force with weight bearing. Mensical tears and premature DJD are not commonly seen until adulthood.

Adult Sequelae
Presenting Symptoms

The adult sequelae of Blount disease have not been well documented. In one study of Swedish adults who had infantile Blount disease, 49 patients with a total of 86 involved lower extremities were evaluated at a mean age of 38 years.[50] The patients had undergone either tibial osteotomy (35 limbs), epiphysiodesis (13 limbs), or no treatment (38 limbs). All limbs had only mild deformity in adulthood. At follow-up, approximately one third of patients had knee pain with ambulation, whereas the rest had no symptoms. Only 11 patients had clinical signs and symptoms of knee joint arthrosis, 9 of whom were graded as having mild symptoms. However, 10 patients had undergone surgery of the medial meniscus at a mean age of 29 years, the sequelae of which is not known. In another study of infantile Blount disease, the authors evaluated 19 limbs in 12 symptomatic adolescents and young adults who had been treated surgically.[51] After arthrotomy or arthroscopy, 12 of 19 knees had evidence of joint arthrosis.

In another Swedish study, the authors evaluated 23 adults (mean age, 47 years) with known late-onset Blount disease.[52] As adolescents, 7 of 23 underwent tibial osteotomy, 11 underwent epiphysiodesis, and 5 underwent no treatment. All patients had only mild genu varum deformities in adulthood. Most were symptom free, with only nine showing early signs of knee arthrosis. At follow-up, no patient had undergone joint arthroplasty. The body mass index of these patients was not recorded.

The association between mild to moderate tibia vara, regardless of the etiology, and the development of knee arthrosis is not well understood. Sharma et al[53] did not report a significantly increased incidence of knee osteoarthritis in patients with varus lower extremity alignment. In contrast, a large, longitudinal cohort study by Brouwer et al[54] showed that varus knee malalignment is associated with the development of radiographic knee osteoarthritis. Other authors have also hypothesized that varus knee alignment and medial sloping of the proximal tibia may predispose patients to progressive DJD.[55,56]

The development and progression of knee osteoarthritis is a complicated scenario that has many etiologies and influences, not all of which are known to the surgeon who is treating end-stage knee DJD. Although Blount disease is not commonly implicated as a causative factor of knee arthritis requiring knee replacement, some patients with tibia vara who develop DJD likely had subclinical Blount disease as children and adolescents. The relatively low incidence of Blount disease, however, compared with the extremely high incidence of idiopathic osteoarthritis in adults, makes it difficult to determine the actual effects of prior Blount disease on the development of later knee arthritis.

Physical Examination

Adults with sequelae of Blount disease may present with concerns about varus knee deformity, instability about the knee, and knee pain with stiffness. The pain may be activity related and mechanical in nature, possibly related to medial meniscus pathology, or chronic, suggesting premature arthrosis. Because Blount disease is sometimes undiagnosed in childhood or adolescence, not all patients will report a history of the disease. If the patient was treated for Blount disease, knowing the complete surgical history and age(s) when the procedures were performed is useful, especially if future surgery is planned.

Observational gait analysis is an important first step in the physical examination. The patient ideally should be evaluated walking toward and away from the examiner in a long hallway or sizeable office space. Gait deviations from pain, knee range of motion during gait, evidence of lateral thrusting of the knee, and rotational malalignment should be evaluated. A careful examination of the entire lower extremity is needed, including evauation of hip, knee, and ankle range of motion, assessment of knee ligament stability, and testing of motor strength and sensory function.

Imaging Studies

Radiographic studies similar to those obtained to assess the patient with an LLD are useful for the adult with sequelae of Blount disease. Bilateral weight-bearing long leg films ranging from the hip to the foot allow assessment of the mechanical axis of the lower limb and identification of other sites of deformity, such as in the distal femur, in addition to the knee in either limb. Evaluation of the lateral radiographs is also critical to assess sagittal malalignment, especially of the tibial plateau, where posterior and posteromedial sloping commonly develop in association with Blount disease. Arthrography of the knee, or MRI with and without intra-articular contrast, are useful to assess the degree of joint incongruity and the need for potential joint-leveling procedures. MRI also helps assess the quality of the articular cartilage and the condition of the menisci.

Interventions for the Adult Patient
Nonsurgical Treatment
For patients with symptoms of early knee DJD and minimal varus deformity, treatment with NSAIDs, strengthening and flexibility, activity modifications, and weight loss may be useful. No study has evaluated knee braces designed to unload the medial compartment for adults with a history of Blount disease; however, some patients will obtain some relief with brace application. In the experience of this chapter's authors, shoe orthotics with lateral posting have been attempted with little success in improving symptoms.

Surgical Treatment
For adults with mechanical knee symptoms, reasonable limb alignment, no knee instability, and imaging consistent with meniscal or mild degenerative knee pathology, arthroscopy may be useful to alleviate symptoms. Débridement of degenerative meniscal tears and assessment of articular cartilage are primarily performed for these carefully selected patients. Careful follow-up is necessary to identify those patients with progressive knee DJD over time and intervene in the future with other modalities when appropriate.

Tibial osteotomy with gradual correction of all aspects of the deformity, including alignment, rotation, and length, is the best option for patients with minimal joint arthrosis at presentation.[44] The techniques described are similar to those used to correct these deformities in older children and adolescents. For those patients with joint line deformity, elevation of the medial tibial plateau also can be performed at the time of the original procedure. A preoperative discussion similar to the one recommended for patients undergoing lengthening procedures is necessary for patients undergoing osteotomies. Pain, prolonged use of an external fixator,

joint stiffness, nerve injury, and infection are some of the important concerns for adults undergoing corrective osteotomies for knee deformities.

Adults with knee DJD and varus knee deformity are best treated using knee realignment and total knee arthroplasty (TKA). Although severe deformities may require staging of the surgery (that is, corrective osteotomy first, followed by TKA), most deformities can be corrected using well-planned osteotomies and modular knee implants during one surgical procedure.[57] This method yields the most reliable results for adults with sequelae of Blount disease. As with any arthroplasty, especially in older individuals, careful preoperative assessment, individualized perioperative medical management, and a comprehensive postoperative rehabilitation program are needed to ensure patient safety and a successful recovery.

Expert Opinion
Patient Evaluation
Careful evaluation of the patient and selection of appropriate treatment modalities are the most important aspects of treating adults with sequelae of Blount disease. Unlike patients with knee osteoarthritis, these patients have limb alignment and intra-articular deformities that are primary components of their disease, not secondary changes. Because of this, nonsurgical modalities are often less efficacious. Patient factors such as smoking, weight, and activity must be addressed before undertaking surgery of any kind for adults with sequelae of Blount disease.

Preferred Interventions
Younger patients with symptoms but little evidence of arthrosis are best treated with corrective osteotomy. In the opinion of this chapter's authors, single-plane deformities with less than 20° of proximal tibial varus without a joint line deformity and a significant LLD are best treated with acute correction, internal fixation, and prophylactic anterior compartment release at the time of surgery. Most other patients, especially those with complex or severe deformities, are treated with gradual correction using an external fixator. Although not as well tolerated by patients as acute correction and internal fixation, gradual fixation allows more complete and anatomic realignment with less risk of compartment syndrome and nerve injury sometimes seen with acute

realignment of large deformities. Patients need to be counseled that successful realignment surgery does not eliminate the possibility that they may develop progressive knee osteoarthritis.

TKA for patients with knee deformity from Blount disease is challenging. The authors of this chapter prefer to perform a single surgery that corrects the deformity using preplanned osteotomies. The implants must also be carefully preselected to ensure that sizing is appropriate, that accommodations can be made for the deformity correction, and that intraoperative adjustments can be easily made. Only patients with severe deformity and advanced knee osteoarthritis require staged limb realignment followed by TKA. The surgeon must be mindful that arthrosis of the hip and ankle may affect outcomes.

Conclusion

LLD is common in adults and may result from several etiologies including traumatic injuries, developmental conditions, and infections that occur in childhood. LLD measuring less than 2 cm generally have little effect on gait and likely do not cause significant problems in adults. Larger discrepancies have been associated with back pain, scoliosis, and hip pain, as well as the development of premature osteoarthritis of the spine and lower limb, although the sequelae of LLD is not completely understood. Shoe lifts are helpful for treating symptoms in patients with small discrepancies. Limb lengthening and limb shortening procedures are options for adults with symptomatic discrepancies. Some discrepancies can be improved by limb lengthening or shortening during total hip replacement. Preoperative patient education about the risks and benefits of limb equalization procedures is critical because these procedures are associated with significant complications.

Little is known about the adult sequelae of Blount disease. For many patients who enter adulthood with minimal knee deformity, painless knee function can be expected at least through middle age. Medial meniscal degeneration is more common in adults who had infantile Blount disease compared with patients who had adolescent disease. Corrective osteotomies are the best choice for the symptomatic adult without advanced knee arthrosis. Knee replacement, with realignment in severe deformities, is the treatment of choice for patients with knee osteoarthritis.

References

1. Woerman AL, Binder-Macleod SA: Leg length discrepancy assessment: Accuracy and precision in five clinical methods of evaluation. *J Orthop Sports Phys Ther* 1984;5(5):230-239.

2. Gross RH: Leg length discrepancy: How much is too much? *Orthopedics* 1978;1(4):307-310.

3. Guichet JM, Spivak JM, Trouilloud P, Grammont PM: Lower limb-length discrepancy: An epidemiologic study. *Clin Orthop Relat Res* 1991(272):235-241.

4. Allen PE, Jenkinson A, Stephens MM, O'Brien T: Abnormalities in the uninvolved lower limb in children with spastic hemiplegia: The effect of actual and functional leg-length discrepancy. *J Pediatr Orthop* 2000;20(1):88-92.

5. Inan M, Chan G, Littleton AG, Kubiak P, Bowen JR: Efficacy and safety of percutaneous epiphysiodesis. *J Pediatr Orthop* 2008;28(6):648-651.

6. Ramseier LE, Sukthankar A, Exner GU: Minimal invasive epiphysiodesis using a modified "Canale" technique for correction of angular deformities and limb leg length discrepancies. *J Child Orthop* 2009;3(1):33-37.

7. Gabriel KR, Crawford AH, Roy DR, True MS, Sauntry S: Percutaneous epiphyseodesis. *J Pediatr Orthop* 1994;14(3):358-362.

8. Porat S, Peyser A, Robin GC: Equalization of lower limbs by epiphysiodesis: Results of treatment. *J Pediatr Orthop* 1991;11(4):442-448.

9. Ogilvie JW, King K: Epiphysiodesis: Two-year clinical results using a new technique. *J Pediatr Orthop* 1990;10(6):809-811.

10. Timperlake RW, Bowen JR, Guille JT, Choi IH: Prospective evaluation of fifty-three consecutive percutaneous epiphysiodeses of the distal femur and proximal tibia and fibula. *J Pediatr Orthop* 1991;11(3):350-357.

11. Blair VP III, Schoenecker PL, Sheridan JJ, Capelli AM: Closed shortening of the femur. *J Bone Joint Surg Am* 1989;71(10):1440-1447.

12. Chapman ME, Duwelius PJ, Bray TJ, Gordon JE: Closed intramedullary femoral osteotomy: Shortening and derotation procedures. *Clin Orthop Relat Res* 1993(287):245-251.

13. Sabharwal S, Green S, McCarthy J, Hamdy RC: What's new in limb lengthening and deformity correction. *J Bone Joint Surg Am* 2011;93(2):213-221.

14. Song KM, Halliday SE, Little DG: The effect of limb-length discrepancy on gait. *J Bone Joint Surg Am* 1997;79(11):1690-1698.

15. Bhave A, Paley D, Herzenberg JE: Improvement in gait parameters after lengthening for the treatment of limb-length discrepancy. *J Bone Joint Surg Am* 1999;81(4):529-534.

16. Kaufman KR, Miller LS, Sutherland DH: Gait asymmetry in patients with limb-length inequality. *J Pediatr Orthop* 1996;16(2):144-150.

17. Soukka A, Alaranta H, Tallroth K, Heliövaara M: Leg-length inequality in people of working age: The association between mild inequality and low-back pain is questionable. *Spine (Phila Pa 1976)* 1991;16(4):429-431.

18. Grundy PF, Roberts CJ: Does unequal leg length cause back pain? A case-control study. *Lancet* 1984;2(8397):256-258.

19. Gofton JP: Persistent low back pain and leg length disparity. *J Rheumatol* 1985;12(4):747-750.

20. Giles LG, Taylor JR: Low-back pain associated with leg length inequality. *Spine (Phila Pa 1976)* 1981;6(5):510-521.

21. Hoikka V, Ylikoski M, Tallroth K: Leg-length inequality has poor correlation with lumbar scoliosis: A radiological study of 100 patients with chronic low-back pain. *Arch Orthop Trauma Surg* 1989;108(3):173-175.

22. Nourbakhsh MR, Arab AM: Relationship between mechanical factors and incidence of low back pain. *J Orthop Sports Phys Ther* 2002;32(9):447-460.

23. Golightly YM, Allen KD, Renner JB, Helmick CG, Salazar A, Jordan JM: Relationship of limb length inequality with radiographic knee and hip osteoarthritis. *Osteoarthritis Cartilage* 2007;15(7):824-829.

24. Tjernström B, Rehnberg L: Back pain and arthralgia before and after lengthening: 75 patients questioned after 6 (1-11) years. *Acta Orthop Scand* 1994;65(3):328-332.

25. Papaioannou T, Stokes I, Kenwright J: Scoliosis associated with limb-length inequality. *J Bone Joint Surg Am* 1982;64(1):59-62.

26. Friberg O: Clinical symptoms and biomechanics of lumbar spine and hip joint in leg length inequality. *Spine (Phila Pa 1976)* 1983;8(6):643-651.

27. Krakovits G: [On the effect of leg shortening on the statics and dynamics of the hip joint]. *Z Orthop Ihre Grenzgeb* 1967;102(3):418-423.

28. Brand RA, Yack HJ: Effects of leg length discrepancies on the forces at the hip joint. *Clin Orthop Relat Res* 1996(333):172-180.

29. Stanitski DF: Limb-length inequality: Assessment and treatment options. *J Am Acad Orthop Surg* 1999;7(3):143-153.

30. Terry MA, Winell JJ, Green DW, et al: Measurement variance in limb length discrepancy: Clinical and radiographic assessment of interobserver and intraobserver variability. *J Pediatr Orthop* 2005;25(2):197-201.

31. Aaron A, Weinstein D, Thickman D, Eilert R: Comparison of orthoroentgenography and computed tomography in the measurement of limb-length discrepancy. *J Bone Joint Surg Am* 1992;74(6):897-902.

32. Hasler CC: [Leg length inequality: Indications for treatment and importance of shortening procedures]. *Orthopade* 2000;29(9):766-774.

33. Eyres KS, Douglas DL, Bell MJ: Closed intramedullary osteotomy for the correction of deformities of the femur. *J R Coll Surg Edinb* 1993;38(5):302-306.

34. Johansson JE, Barrington TW: Femoral shortening by a step-cut osteotomy for leg-length discrepancy in adults. *Clin Orthop Relat Res* 1983(181):132-136.

35. Coppola C, Maffulli N: Limb shortening for the management of leg length discrepancy. *J R Coll Surg Edinb* 1999;44(1):46-54.

36. Gulsen M, Ozkan C: Angular shortening and delayed gradual distraction for the treatment of asymmetrical bone and soft tissue defects of tibia: a case series. *J Trauma* 2009;66(5):E61-E66.

37. Nordsletten L, Holm I, Steen H, Bjerkreim I: Muscle function after femoral shortening osteotomies at the subtrochanteric and mid-diaphyseal level: A follow-up study. *Arch Orthop Trauma Surg* 1994;114(1):37-39.

38. Kempf I, Grosse A, Abalo C: Locked intramedullary nailing: Its application to femoral and tibial axial, rotational, lengthening, and shortening osteotomies. *Clin Orthop Relat Res* 1986(212):165-173.

39. Dahl MT, Gulli B, Berg T: Complications of limb lengthening: A learning curve. *Clin Orthop Relat Res* 1994(301):10-18.

40. Eberson CP, Hogan KA, Moore DC, Ehrlich MG: Effect of low-intensity ultrasound stimulation on consolidation of the regenerate zone in a rat model of distraction osteogenesis. *J Pediatr Orthop* 2003;23(1):46-51.

41. Chen F, Hui JH, Chan WK, Lee EH: Cultured mesenchymal stem cell transfers in the treatment of partial

growth arrest. *J Pediatr Orthop* 2003;23(4): 425-429.

42. Schmalzried TP, Amstutz HC, Dorey FJ: Nerve palsy associated with total hip replacement: Risk factors and prognosis. *J Bone Joint Surg Am* 1991;73(7):1074-1080.

43. Eggli S, Hankemayer S, Müller ME: Nerve palsy after leg lengthening in total replacement arthroplasty for developmental dysplasia of the hip. *J Bone Joint Surg Br* 1999;81(5):843-845.

44. Sabharwal S, Zhao C, McClemens E: Correlation of body mass index and radiographic deformities in children with Blount disease. *J Bone Joint Surg Am* 2007;89(6):1275-1283.

45. Raney EM, Topoleski TA, Yaghoubian R, Guidera KJ, Marshall JG: Orthotic treatment of infantile tibia vara. *J Pediatr Orthop* 1998;18(5):670-674.

46. Castañeda P, Urquhart B, Sullivan E, Haynes RJ: Hemiepiphysiodesis for the correction of angular deformity about the knee. *J Pediatr Orthop* 2008;28(2):188-191.

47. Feldman DS, Madan SS, Ruchelsman DE, Sala DA, Lehman WB: Accuracy of correction of tibia vara: Acute versus gradual correction. *J Pediatr Orthop* 2006;26(6):794-798.

48. Gordon JE, Heidenreich FP, Carpenter CJ, Kelly-Hahn J, Schoenecker PL: Comprehensive treatment of late-onset tibia vara. *J Bone Joint Surg Am* 2005;87(7):1561-1570.

49. McCarthy JJ, Mark AK, Davidson RS: Treatment of angular deformities of the tibia in children: Acute versus gradual correction. *J Surg Orthop Adv* 2007;16(3): 118-122.

50. Ingvarsson T, Hägglund G, Ramgren B, Jonsson K, Zayer M: Long-term results after infantile Blount's disease. *J Pediatr Orthop B* 1998;7(3):226-229.

51. Hofmann A, Jones RE, Herring JA: Blount's disease after skeletal maturity. *J Bone Joint Surg Am* 1982;64(7): 1004-1009.

52. Ingvarsson T, Hägglund G, Ramgren B, Jonsson K, Zayer M: Long-term results after adolescent Blount's disease. *J Pediatr Orthop B* 1997;6(2):153-156.

53. Sharma L, Song J, Felson DT, Cahue S, Shamiyeh E, Dunlop DD: The role of knee alignment in disease progression and functional decline in knee osteoarthritis. *JAMA* 2001;286(2):188-195.

54. Brouwer GM, van Tol AW, Bergink AP, et al: Association between valgus and varus alignment and the development and progression of radiographic osteoarthritis of the knee. *Arthritis Rheum* 2007;56(4):1204-1211.

55. Cerejo R, Dunlop DD, Cahue S, Channin D, Song J, Sharma L: The influence of alignment on risk of knee osteoarthritis progression according to baseline stage of disease. *Arthritis Rheum* 2002;46(10):2632-2636.

56. Cooke TD, Pichora D, Siu D, Scudamore RA, Bryant JT: Surgical implications of varus deformity of the knee with obliquity of joint surfaces. *J Bone Joint Surg Br* 1989;71(4):560-565.

57. Teeny SM, Krackow KA, Hungerford DS, Jones M: Primary total knee arthroplasty in patients with severe varus deformity: A comparative study. *Clin Orthop Relat Res* 1991(273):19-31.

CHAPTER 9

DOWN SYNDROME

PETER D. PIZZUTILLO, MD

INTRODUCTION

The facial appearance of children and adults with mongolism, now known as Down syndrome, has been observed in individuals of all races.[1] More than 50 years ago, Lejeune et al[2] reported the presence of an extra chromosome, chromosome 21, in the karyotype of individuals with Down syndrome. Although earlier reports noted a clinical association between advanced maternal age and Down syndrome, the current practice of prenatal studies of at-risk pregnancies in older mothers with the option of termination of pregnancy has resulted in a younger profile of parents.[3] Trisomy 21 occurs in 1 liveborn infant per 600; it results in various clinical expressions and is the most common cause of mental retardation.

Recent technologic advances have allowed more than 300 identified genes to be sequenced in chromosome 21, the smallest human autosome. The broad spectrum of clinical issues and phenotypic expression as well as the various degrees of involvement in these individuals may be the result of direct or indirect interactions with other genes or gene products.[4-6] Investigators continue to decipher the genetic base of affected individuals with the hope of discovering effective interventions that may delay the onset of degenerative problems and substantially improve their quality of life.

COMMON PROBLEMS AND CHILDHOOD INTERVENTIONS

Infants with Down syndrome are usually identified at birth as the result of prenatal studies or on the basis of observation of typical physical findings that are confirmed by chromosomal analysis. The early diagnosis of serious clinical problems, such as cardiac anomalies and thyroid dysfunction, has allowed for treatment during the neonatal period that significantly improves patient outcome. Other health issues may develop with increasing age, including delayed motor development, obstructive sleep apnea, obesity, and varying degrees of cognitive impairment.[7,8] Musculoskeletal conditions that may be observed in the first and second decades of life include patellar and hip joint instability, slipped capital femoral epiphysis (SCFE), bunion formation, and cervical instability.[9]

OUTCOMES: NATURAL HISTORY AND RESULTS OF INTERVENTIONS

Without appropriate intervention, many infants with Down syndrome would succumb to significant cardiac anomalies that would hamper growth and development and severely limit activity level and longevity. Thyroid dysfunction that persists without treatment results in

Dr. Pizzutillo or an immediate family member serves as a board member, owner, officer, or committee member of the American Academy of Orthopaedic Surgeons.

FIGURE 1

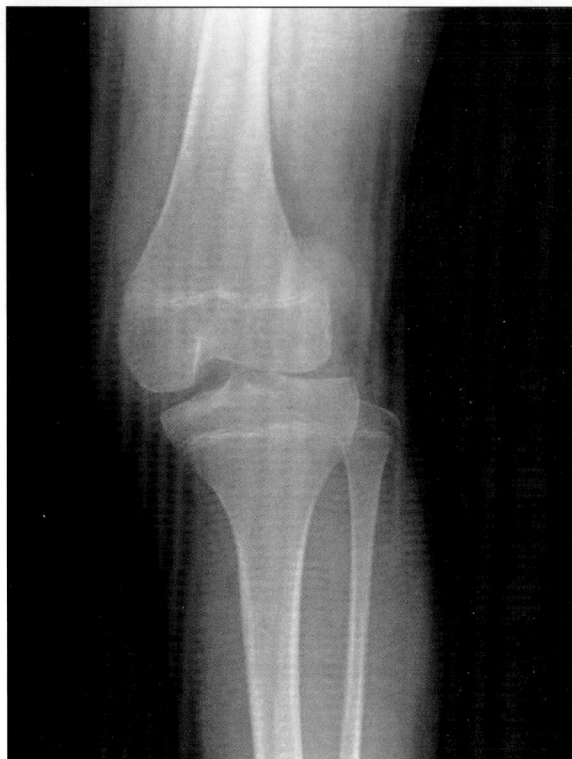

Supine AP radiograph of the knee joint reveals significant lateral patellar displacement.

major cognitive, growth, and motor impairment. Advances in neonatal screening and medical/surgical interventions have allowed early diagnosis and effective management of cardiac anomalies and thyroid disease that have significantly improved overall development and growth.

Motor development in children with Down syndrome does not progress in the same manner as in unaffected children. The cause of the delay is unknown and has been attributed to low muscle tone, general ligamentous laxity, or central nervous system dysfunction. With neurologic maturation, the delay in motor function may improve to a level that allows many individuals to fully participate in complex motor activities, including athletic endeavors.[10] Interventions to improve cognitive deficits have not yet been shown to result in significant improvement.[11,12]

The failure to recognize cervical instability and myelopathy, patellar instability, and hip joint instability in children with Down syndrome results in serious impairment and diminished overall function. In these children, quality of life is negatively affected and the burden of care on family and society is increased. Late recognition and treatment of these problems are not likely to have the same benefits as when treated early in life.

Orthopaedic conditions manifest differently in those with Down syndrome than in unaffected individuals. Whether this difference is due to factors at the cellular level, qualitative alterations of neuromuscular control, or gross anatomic variations is unknown; however, recognizing that intrinsic differences exist that may affect evaluation and treatment is important. This finding is especially evident in the evaluation and treatment of cervical spine instability

Patellar Instability

Patellar instability occurs more often in the adolescent and the adult with Down syndrome and is likely due to ligamentous laxity and dysplasia of the distal femoral condyles (**Figure 1**). When acute patellar dislocation occurs in individuals with Down syndrome, it is not usually associated with hemarthrosis, disruption of the medial retinaculum and the medial patellofemoral ligament, or intra-articular fracture of the knee.[13] Spontaneous patellar reduction typically occurs and treatment should be focused on bracing and physical therapy. When patellar instability persists despite these interventions, the realignment of proximal and distal soft tissues successfully eliminates or substantially reduces the incidence of instability. With severe ligamentous laxity, redislocation is likely and stable patellar excursion may be enhanced by reconstruction of the medial retinaculum or the medial patellofemoral ligament. In the skeletally mature knee, the tibial tuberosity may be reoriented to improve the vector forces delivered through the patellar tendon in the presence of an increased Q angle, but it is not frequently required.[14]

Hip Subluxation and Dislocation

Atraumatic hip subluxation or dislocation may occur at any age in individuals with Down syndrome. Spontaneous dislocation has been associated with ligamentous laxity and hypotonia; however, other unknown factors

FIGURE 2

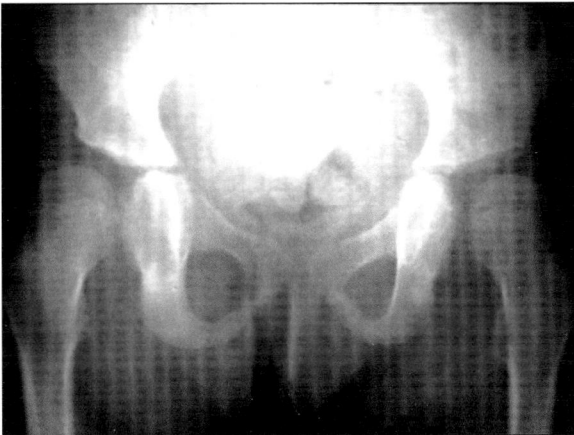

Supine AP radiograph of the hips and pelvis of a child with Down syndrome shows spontaneous painless hip instability.

may be in effect.[15] Spontaneous reduction is the rule in the young patient; surgical reduction is rarely needed. Dislocation and reduction may be observed in one or both hips and felt continuously in flexion and extension. Although this dislocation is disconcerting to caretakers, the affected child usually does not experience pain or problems with perineal care or ambulation.

Hip instability that develops in early childhood or during adolescence may require treatment that includes observation, bracing, or surgical procedures (**Figure 2**). Bracing does not usually result in restoration of hip stability but may decrease the incidence of dislocations. Surgical intervention varies and usually involves reorientation of the proximal femur, imbrication of the hip joint capsule, and realignment of the acetabulum. Unfortunately, the multiple surgical treatments recommended to restore hip stability have not been uniformly successful. Persistent hip subluxation or dislocation are challenging to treat. Hip joint degeneration may be observed after the third decade of life and results in significant pain with weight bearing and impairment of the individual's ambulation.[16]

Slipped Capital Femoral Epiphysis

In the general population, SCFE has been associated with obesity and hypothyroidism. Both obesity and thyroid dysfunction occur with increased incidence in indi-

viduals with Down syndrome and may contribute to the increased incidence of SCFE in this population.[17] SCFE in individuals with Down syndrome has been treated with the same surgical techniques that have been used in the general population with SCFE. Despite similar surgical interventions, individuals with Down syndrome and SCFE have experienced a higher complication rate, including osteonecrosis of the femoral head, progressive deformity, and chondrolysis with hip joint degeneration. The factors that contribute to increased morbidity are unknown. Whether differences in intrinsic biology or specific surgical interventions are responsible for the difference in outcomes in this population is also unknown.

Hallux Valgus

Hallux valgus with bunion formation may be observed in adolescents and is likely a result of hyperpronation of the flexible pes planus and muscle imbalance. Orthotic intervention in the early stages of bunion development has been recommended to prevent progression to severe deformity but has not yet proved to be efficacious. Surgical correction of bunions in the skeletally immature patient with Down syndrome has produced only fair results with a high likelihood of recurrent deformity. Recent trends in treatment of the adolescent with symptomatic bunions have favored orthotic treatment and shoe modification rather than surgical intervention.

Cervical Instability

The most serious clinical condition in individuals with Down syndrome is the development of cervical instability with the potential for cervical stenosis, myelopathy, and radiculopathy. Increased mobility at the atlantoaxial junction, reported by Spitzer et al,[18] and at the occipitocervical junction, reported by Tredwell et al,[19] has been observed in 20% of individuals with Down syndrome. Over the past 5 decades, observations of radiographic changes of the cervical spine in patients with Down syndrome have revealed no greater insight into factors that could result in increased intersegmental mobility or instability. Pueschel et al[20] reported that the radiographic appearance of the cervical spine in individuals with Down syndrome is different than in unaffected individuals. Criteria to evaluate cervical spine instability have been developed from the study of radiographs of the general population; however, they are not appropriately applied in the evaluation of instability in individuals with Down syndrome. Neutral lateral flexion and extension radiographs of the cervical spine have been the primary mode of imaging evaluation for those with Down syndrome. Cristofaro et al[21] applied the radiographic criteria derived from the population without Down syndrome and observed that 20% of those with Down syndrome had atlantoaxial instability and at least 20% had occipitocervical instability. Among individuals with Down syndrome who have been followed into adulthood, 33% exhibited radiographic abnormalities, yet only 3% developed neurologic problems.[21]

Recognizing the differences that exist between the radiographs of the general population and those of the population with Down syndrome is important. To be clinically relevant, radiographic criteria of cervical spine instability in individuals with Down syndrome must be correlated with the clinical conditions. This concept results in a significant shift in the understanding of instability and requires language that more accurately reflects the clinical reality. Abnormalities on radiographs of the general population that suggest cervical spine instability frequently have little clinical correlation in the population with Down syndrome and may be more appropriately indicative of hypermobility rather than instability.

Hypermobility refers to the radiographic appearance of increased motion at cervical segments in flexion and extension. In individuals without Down syndrome, increased motion correlates with clinical conditions such as ligamentous injury that are associated with neurologic impairment, whereas clinical associations have not been established in the population with Down syndrome. Instability suggests a more severe degree of intersegmental motion that threatens the integrity of the spinal cord and the nerve roots. Early experience in the evaluation of cervical spine radiographs in patients with Down syndrome frequently resulted in a diagnosis of cervical instability and prophylactic surgical stabilization of the spine in the absence of clinical signs and symptoms. Davidson[22] reported that only a small group of individuals with Down syndrome developed neurologic compromise as a result of cervical instability and will require surgical stabilization.

In individuals with Down syndrome, hypermobility more accurately describes changes seen on routine cervical spine images in relation to associated clinical conditions than does instability. The term hypermobility is not used to diminish concern regarding the development of cervical instability or to decrease the awareness that neurologic compromise may occur in the individual with Down syndrome. Neurologic compromise usually is a result of atlantoaxial instability or occipitocervical instability in association with bony anomalies of the base of the skull (for example, basilar impression) or of the upper cervical spine (for example, atlantal arch hypoplasia).[23]

Because decreased physical tolerance is the earliest sign of impending myelopathy resulting from cervical instability, educating patients and their parents about how to identify a significant decrease in physical vigor and report it immediately to their physician is important. Patients with cardiac and thyroid dysfunction also may present with diminished physical endurance and require specific evaluation.

ADULT SEQUELAE
Presenting Symptoms
At routine evaluation, adults with Down syndrome may present with no problems or with reports of diminished physical energy, unsteady gait, or unwillingness to ambulate. The comprehensive evaluation of these symptoms includes investigation of cardiac disorders, thyroid dysfunction, neurologic compromise, and orthopaedic conditions because each of these systemic issues may have a similar presentation.

Evaluation
Physical Examination
Physical examination of the adult with Down syndrome should be comprehensive to evaluate for cardiac disease and hypothyroidism, alterations in memory and cognition, and visual impairment. Advances in the medical care of individuals with Down syndrome have resulted in improved quality of life and a significant increase in longevity that may span into the eighth decade. Individuals with and without Down syndrome have the same general health problems as they age; however, patients older than 50 years with Down syndrome have a higher incidence of seizure disorder, and those older than 60 years have a higher incidence of dementia.

Orthopaedic examination includes the evaluation of head and neck posture, spinal alignment, and extremity function as well as the determination of neurologic integrity. Qualitative gait evaluation of the barefoot individual wearing shorts provides helpful clues to identification of clinical issues involving foot placement, leg alignment, stride, stability, and limp. Special attention should be given to the range of motion and stability of the hip and knee joints. Subluxation and degenerative disease of the hip joint will result in limited hip motion in abduction and internal rotation with subsequent painful weight bearing on the involved limb.

Knee malalignment, painful knee joint motion, and patellar subluxation/dislocation occur frequently in this population and demand specific attention. Instability of the knee joint ligaments is not common despite the presence of generalized ligamentous laxity and hypotonia.

Imaging Studies

A recent history of diminished physical endurance, even with normal neurologic findings, suggests the need for lateral flexion and extension radiographs of the cervical spine as well as radiographic evaluation of the hip and knee joints.

Cervical spine radiographs may reveal hypermobility or instability at the atlantoaxial or occipitocervical junction, disk degeneration, osteophyte formation, foraminal encroachment, arthritic facet joints, or narrowing of the spinal canal.[24] In addition, radiographs may demonstrate os odontoideum or abnormal ossification of the atlantal arch.

Cervical spine MRI best demonstrates any compromise of the space available for the cord resulting from hypertrophied soft tissue within the spinal canal, as well as signal intensity changes within the cord consistent with early myelopathy and degenerative clefts within the cord resulting from long-standing instability. Flexion and extension MRIs may demonstrate cervical cord impingement with signal intensity changes within the cord in long-standing instability but not with recent onset of instability.

Hip radiographs may reveal subluxation with varying degrees of hip joint arthritis or degenerative collapse of the femoral head. Rapid progression of arthritic changes in the hip joint may occur in periods as short as 1 year. Knee radiographs may demonstrate arthritic changes involving the three compartments of the knee joint,

patellar instability, and distal femoral dysplasia. For the patient with impaired gait, weight-bearing radiographs of the feet aid in the identification of pathology such as severe hallux valgus and arthritis of the metatarsophalangeal joints.

INTERVENTIONS FOR THE ADULT PATIENT

Cervical Spine

Instability of the occipitocervical or the atlantoaxial junction is not a frequent clinical problem in the adult with Down syndrome. When instability is present, surgical stabilization with internal fixation is indicated to preserve neurologic function (**Figure 3**). Absolute bony or soft-tissue stenosis of the cervical canal, as documented on MRI, may require decompressive laminectomy with or without stabilization. In Davidson's[22] review of adults with Down syndrome, 33% exhibited radiographic evidence of degenerative changes of the cervical spine (**Figure 4**) but only 3% developed neurologic problems. Treatment of this population must be focused on the patient and their clinical findings and not on radiographic abnormalities.

Hip Joint

Symptomatic degenerative changes of the hip joint are rarely responsive to nonsurgical interventions such as physical therapy or assisted ambulation (**Figure 5**). Disease progression results in significant restriction in ambulation, and ultimately, loss of ambulation because of pain. Surgical interventions include periacetabular osteotomy,[25] Chiari pelvic osteotomy, total hip arthroplasty, and hip arthrodesis. The decision for surgical intervention should be made on an individual basis. The wide spectrum of cognitive and motor impairment in this population and the existence of comorbidities such as diabetes mellitus, marked obesity, and advanced cardiac or pulmonary compromise are important factors in the decision-making process. The individual in relatively good health who is actively involved in the home or residential environment is likely a good candidate for total hip arthroplasty. Generalized ligamentous laxity, poor muscle tone, inability to cooperate with a postoperative therapy program, or a residential environment that increases the risk of postoperative infection might suggest a salvage procedure, such as arthrodesis of the

FIGURE 3

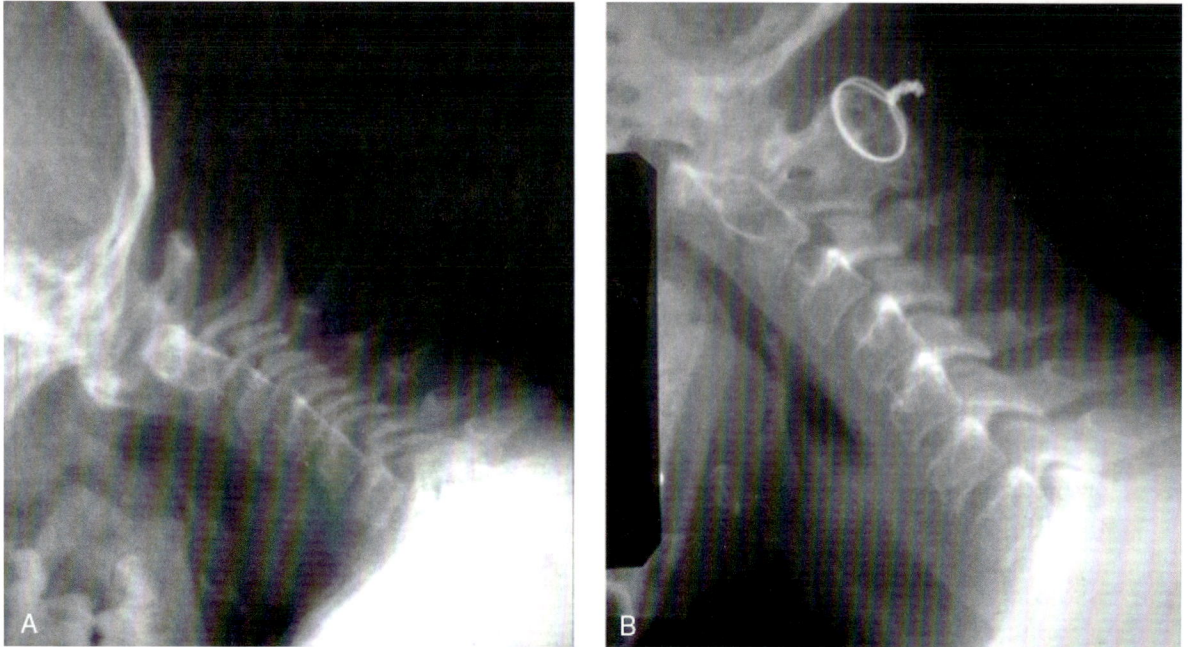

Lateral flexion radiographs in a patient who was treated with C1-C2 surgical fusion. **A,** Preoperative view shows atlantoaxial instability. **B,** Postoperative view.

FIGURE 4

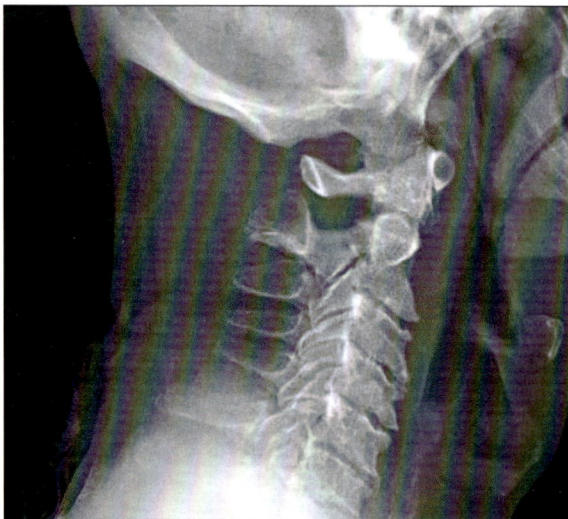

Lateral radiograph of the cervical spine in an adult with Down syndrome demonstrates degenerative changes of the disk and facet joints.

FIGURE 5

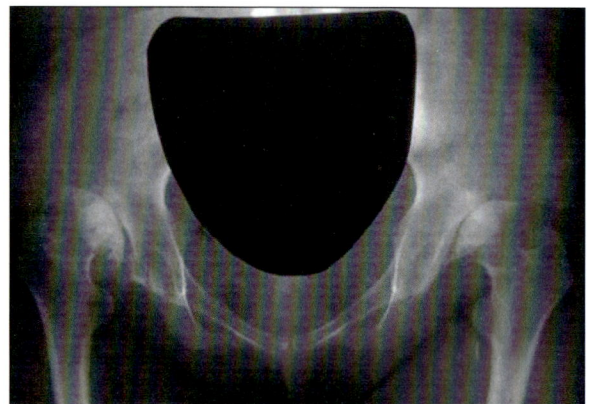

AP weight-bearing radiograph of the hips in an adult with Down syndrome with documented progressive instability demonstrates significant degenerative changes of the hips.

hip, which would not require rigorous rehabilitation, or nonsurgical treatment that essentially relegates the individual to wheelchair ambulation.

Knee Joint

Patellar instability without significant arthritic changes may be treated with physical therapy and an appropriate patellar restraining brace. When nonsurgical techniques are unsuccessful, surgical realignment of the patellofemoral mechanism is indicated. The specific surgical intervention is determined by considering the same physical factors that affect the general population and may include proximal and distal soft-tissue realignment, tendon augmentation of the medial patellofemoral ligament, and bony realignment of the proximal tibia.

Severe arthritic changes in the knee joint require assessment of the same confounding factors that influence the decision-making process for hip joint disorders. In the experience of this chapter's author, surgical intervention for knee arthritis is infrequent in individuals with Down syndrome.

Foot

Pes planus is common in patients with Down syndrome and is usually asymptomatic. With symptomatic hyperpronation of the foot, orthotic management is successful and is considered the standard of care. Surgical intervention is rarely indicated. Hallux valgus and bunion formation are exacerbated by ligamentous laxity and hyperpronation of the foot. Orthotic support is successful in relieving foot discomfort and providing a more stable foot placement in stance. In the case of intractable discomfort, custom-molded shoes or surgical treatment of hallux valgus and bunions are effective interventions.

CONCLUSION

Improved medical care has resulted in improved quality of life and increased longevity for individuals with Down syndrome. Many individuals continue to live in their family homes and function well, with little to moderate guidance needed. Clinical issues involving the cervical spine, the hip and knee joints, and the feet may adversely affect quality of life and impair function and independence. Many of these clinical problems may be successfully treated with early intervention to preserve function and comfort. Annual clinical evaluation of the

adult with Down syndrome is recommended to better define the natural history of musculoskeletal problems in this population, to allow for early detection of disorders, and to provide more successful intervention.

REFERENCES

1. Down JL: Observations on an ethnic classification of idiots. *Lond Hosp Clin Lect Rep* 1866;3:259-262.
2. Lejeune J, Gautier M, Turpin R: Etude des chromosomes somatiques de neuf enfants mongoliens. *C R Hebd Seances Acad Sci* 1959;248(11):1721-1722.
3. Egan JF, Benn PA, Zelop CM, Bolnick A, Gianferrari E, Borgida AF: Down syndrome births in the United States from 1989 to 2001. *Am J Obstet Gynecol* 2004;191(3):1044-1048.
4. Lyle R, Béna F, Gagos S, et al: Genotype-phenotype correlations in Down syndrome identified by array CGH in 30 cases of partial trisomy and partial monosomy chromosome 21. *Eur J Hum Genet* 2009;17(4):454-466.
5. Hattori M, Fujiyama A, Taylor TD, et al: Chromosome 21 mapping and sequencing consortium: The DNA sequence of human chromosome 21. *Nature* 2000;405(6784):311-319.
6. Aït Yahya-Graison E, Aubert J, Dauphinot L, et al: Classification of human chromosome 21 gene-expression variations in Down syndrome: Impact on disease phenotypes. *Am J Hum Genet* 2007;81(3):475-491.
7. Murphy J, Hoey HM, Philip M, et al: Guidelines for the medical management of Irish children and adolescents with Down syndrome. *Ir Med J* 2005;98(2):48-52.
8. Ng DK, Chan CH: Obesity is an important risk factor for sleep disordered breathing in children with Down syndrome. *Sleep* 2004;27(5):1023-1024, 1025.
9. Pizzutillo PD, Herman MJ: Musculoskeletal concerns in the young athlete with Down syndrome. *Oper Tech Sports Med* 2006;14:135-141.
10. Dolva AS, Coster W, Lilja M: Functional performance in children with Down syndrome. *Am J Occup Ther* 2004;58(6):621-629.
11. Weathers C: Effects of nutritional supplementation on IQ and certain other variables associated with Down syndrome. *Am J Ment Defic* 1983;88(2):214-217.
12. Ellis JM, Tan HK, Gilbert RE, et al: Supplementation with antioxidants and folinic acid for children with Down's syndrome: Randomised controlled trial. *BMJ* 2008;336(7644):594-597.

13. Dugdale TW, Renshaw TS: Instability of the patello-femoral joint in Down syndrome. *J Bone Joint Surg Am* 1986;68(3):405-413.

14. Mendez AA, Keret D, MacEwen GD: Treatment of patellofemoral instability in Down's syndrome. *Clin Orthop Relat Res* 1988(234):148-158.

15. Bennet GC, Rang M, Roye DP, Aprin H: Dislocation of the hip in trisomy 21. *J Bone Joint Surg Br* 1982;64(3):289-294.

16. Hresko MT, McCarthy JC, Goldberg MJ: Hip disease in adults with Down syndrome. *J Bone Joint Surg Br* 1993;75(4):604-607.

17. Dietz FR, Albanese SA, Katz DA, et al: Slipped capital femoral epiphysis in down syndrome. *J Pediatr Orthop* 2004;24(5):508-513.

18. Spitzer R, Rabinowitch JY, Wybar KC: A study of the abnormalities of the skull, teeth and lenses in mongolism. *Can Med Assoc J* 1961;84(11):567-572.

19. Tredwell SJ, Newman DE, Lockitch G: Instability of the upper cervical spine in Down syndrome. *J Pediatr Orthop* 1990;10(5):602-606.

20. Pueschel SM, Findley TW, Furia J, Gallagher PL, Scola FH, Pezzullo JC: Atlantoaxial instability in Down syndrome: Roentgenographic, neurologic, and somatosensory evoked potential studies. *J Pediatr* 1987;110(4):515-521.

21. Cristofaro HA, Donovan R, Cristofaro J: Orthopaedic abnormalities in an adult population with Down syndrome. *Orthop Tran* 1986;10:442-443.

22. Davidson RG: Atlantoaxial instability in individuals with Down syndrome: A fresh look at the evidence. *Pediatrics* 1988;81(6):857-865.

23. Crockard HA, Stevens JM: Craniovertebral junction anomalies in inherited disorders: Part of the syndrome or caused by the disorder? *Eur J Pediatr* 1995;154(7):504-512.

24. Olive PM, Whitecloud TS III, Bennett JT: Lower cervical spondylosis and myelopathy in adults with Down's syndrome. *Spine (Phila Pa 1976)* 1988;13(7):781-784.

25. Katz DA, Kim YJ, Millis MB: Periacetabular osteotomy in patients with Down's syndrome. *J Bone Joint Surg Br* 2005;87(4):544-547.

INDEX

Page numbers followed by *f* indicate figures; page numbers followed by *t* indicate tables.

T

Talar head beaking, 67, 68

Talocalcaneal coalition, 69

Talocalcaneal resection, indications for, 68

Tanner classification of secondary sexual characteristics, 52*t*

Tarsal coalition, 67–70

Teleoradiography, 91, 91*f*

THA. See Total hip arthroplasty

Thoracic curve decrease, 3

Thoracolumbar/lumbar curve decrease, 3–4

Thoracolumbosacral orthosis, 2

Thyroid dysfunction, 103

Tibial osteotomies, 96–97, 97*f*, 99

Tibial shortening, 92

Tönnis roof angle, 17

Total hip arthroplasty (THA), 13, 15, 93–94
     developmental dysplasia of the hip and, 33, 37, 41

Total knee arthroplasty, 98, 99–100

Trendelenburg gait, 93

Transforaminal lumbar interbody fusion (TLIF), 6, 7, 8

Transphyseal reconstruction, 50

Triphasic bone scanning, 68

Triple arthrodesis, 65, 68, 69

Triple pelvic osteotomy, 15

Trisomy 21, 103

U

UCBL. *See* University of California Biomechanics Laboratory

Ulnar osteotomy, 79, 80

Ulnar deformity, overcorrection of, 79

Ulnar fracture, 78

Unilateral developmental dysplasia of the hip, 35

Unilateral extensor hallucis longus weakness, 3

University of California Biomechanics Laboratory (UCBL) orthoses, 68, 70

Upper extremity conditions. *See* Lateral condyle fractures; Monteggia fracture-dislocation; Supracondylar fractures

V

Valgus elbow, 78

Valgus hindfoot, 63

Valgus posture, 69

Valgus osteotomy, 73

W

Wilson test, 46

Wiltse-Newman classification of spondylolisthesis, 1